D0394329

The Mindful Way *through* Pregnancy

The Mindful Way *through* Pregnancy

MEDITATION, YOGA, AND JOURNALING FOR EXPECTANT MOTHERS

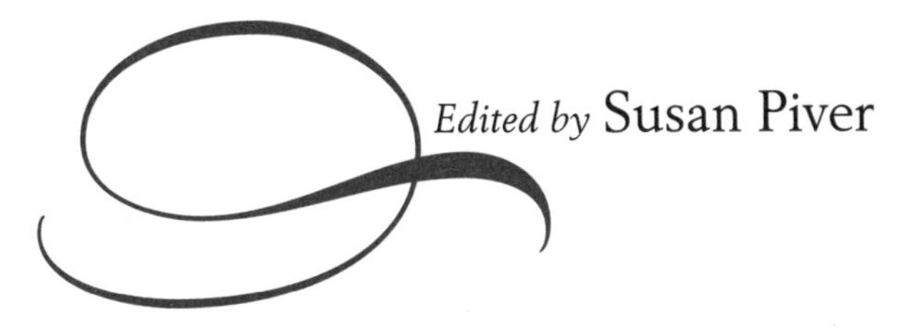

Edited by Susan Piver

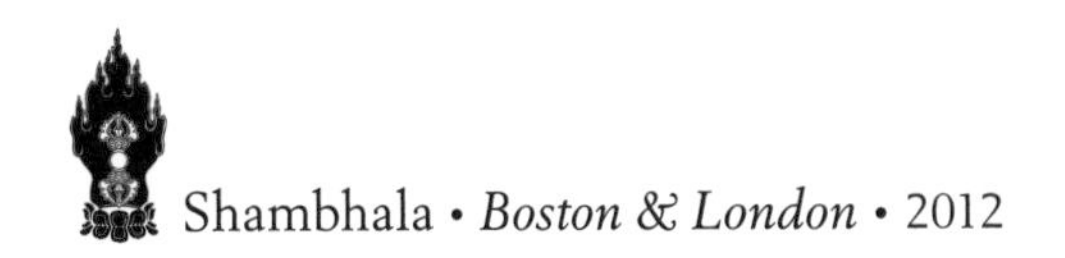

Shambhala • *Boston & London* • 2012

Note: If you have a serious injury or illness, consult a health professional before practicing yoga. Not all exercises and poses are suitable for everyone. This or any exercise can result in injury. To reduce the risk of injury, do not force or cause strain in a yoga pose. When in doubt, consult your health professional.

Shambhala Publications, Inc.
Horticultural Hall
300 Massachusetts Avenue
Boston, Massachusetts 02115
www.shambhala.com

This is a revised edition of a book previously published as *Joyful Birth* (2002).

9 8 7 6 5 4 3 2 1

Printed in China
♾ This edition is printed on acid-free paper that meets the
American National Standards Institute Z39.48 Standard.
♻ Shambhala Publications makes every effort to print on recycled paper.
For more information please visit www.shambhala.com.
Distributed in the United States by Random House, Inc.,
and in Canada by Random House of Canada Ltd

Designed by James D. Skatges

Library of Congress Cataloging-in-Publication Data

The mindful way through pregnancy: meditation, yoga, and journaling
for expectant mothers / edited by Susan Piver.—1st Shambhala ed.
p. cm.
Includes bibliographical references.
ISBN 978-1-59030-966-7 (hardcover with CD)
1. Pregnancy. 2. Self-care, Health. 3. Meditation—Therapeutic use.
I. Piver, Susan, 1957–
RG551.M56 2012
618.2'44—dc23
2011046577

To Carol Hanna and Allison Margaret

Contents

Acknowledgments

Thank you: Robert Bosnak, Duncan Browne, Anne Cushman, Kath Delaney, Amy Fox, Jeniffer Cogliantry, Myla Kabat-Zinn, Joshua Leeds, Greg McCleary, Louise Piver, Zea Piver, David Reich, Elizabeth Rubin, Jill Satterfield, Eden Steinberg, Celia Straus, Stephanie Tade, Geof Thurber.

Introduction

Even as I hold you, I am letting go.
—Alice Walker

When we become pregnant, we receive a great deal of medical, dietary, and lifestyle advice. Of course, it is crucial to pay attention to what we eat, the stages of our baby's development, and how to stay healthy throughout pregnancy. But we can also pay attention to something else: Within the rush of doctor's visits, changes in our bodies, and shopping trips for maternity clothes, a miracle is occurring. Our bodies are giving rise to life. Our hearts are expanding till we fear they may break. Our identities are shifting and changing. Suddenly, perfectly, irrevocably, we are displaced from the center of our own life. With gentleness, we can also explore these aspects of our pregnancy.

The Mindful Way through Pregnancy invites you to slow down, relax, and cherish this magical and momentous time of life. It features illuminating essays written by experts on mindfulness, spirituality, and parenting. This book and CD also offer step-by-step instruction in yoga, meditation, journaling, and more, to help you make the most out of this experience and prepare yourself for childbirth and beyond.

Our culture places extraordinarily high expectations on mothers, expectations that, unquestioned, can rob us of the true joy of pregnancy and motherhood. We are given images of pregnancy as largely a time of happiness, interrupted perhaps by some pesky morning sickness. We expect to feel loving, nurturing, accepting, and fulfilled. Yet often our experience is more complicated. In addition to love and happiness, we may also experience doubt, irritation, and fear. We may find ourselves asking troubling questions about personal identity, relationships, our ability to parent well. *The Mindful Way through Pregnancy* contains exercises and practices to help us slow down, settle in, and relax with our questions and experiences. Here, mindfulness doesn't necessarily mean peacefulness. It refers instead to the willingness to be with ourselves as we are from moment to moment, whether that self is the picture of blissful maternity or of something a bit more, say, cranky or fearful. The material in this book is about embracing the experience of pregnancy—and as with all embraces, it begins with opening, which is a synonym for mindfulness.

As your child grows within you, so does the parent you are to become. Pregnancy is a chance to give birth to yourself as a parent. This book features exercises to help you set intentions for yourself as a mother, examine your values, and think about the kind of relationship you want with your child.

Of course, above almost anything else, pregnancy is a powerful physical event. So, in addition to recommending ways to work with your inner experience, this book offers basic yoga postures to help relax your body, release tension, and prepare for labor.

The CD included with this book features guided meditations to help you achieve deep relaxation, bond with your baby, truly open your heart to motherhood, and more. These meditations can be used during pregnancy and after giving birth. They provide simple ways to relax anytime—something invaluable both during the stresses of pregnancy and afterward.

I hope you'll find the writings and practices in this book helpful as you embark on one of life's most precious and rich experiences.

> *The moment I found out I was pregnant, all I wanted to do was envelop myself in beauty and true nourishment. I was moved to create an environment in which I could focus pure love into this being inside of me. It had nothing to do with the mind. It wasn't a choice or a thought. I was just overflowing with devotion for this being.*
>
> —Zea

I knew that parenting would change my life in ways that I couldn't even dream of. But I assumed that motherhood would start once my baby was out and in my arms. What I didn't understand was that from the moment I opened my heart to the tiny person growing inside me, I would already be a mother.

1

Riding the Waves

Anne Cushman

When I got pregnant for the first time, I was thirty-five years old. I had spent much of the last three years on a pilgrimage all over India, researching a guidebook to ashrams, meditation centers, yoga schools, and sacred sites from the Himalayas to the Arabian Sea. Now I was casting about for another spiritual adventure: Should I return to India to research the history of yoga? Travel to Vietnam to visit my Buddhist teacher's monasteries and my soldier father's battle sites? Go on a three-month Vipassana meditation retreat? But instead, I embarked on a journey I felt would be even more challenging and transformative. I decided to have a baby.

I knew that parenting would change my life in ways I couldn't even dream of. But I assumed that motherhood would start once my baby was out and in my arms. What I didn't understand was that from the moment I opened my heart to the tiny person growing inside me, I would already be a mother. My body and mind would begin a seismic rearrangement, reordering their priorities on every level—hormonal, biochemical, nutritional, emotional—according to the needs of another creature. On a cellular level, I would fall in love. And in doing so, I would open myself to both joy and grief on a scale I had never imagined.

Over the next two years, I carried two babies to term. My first pregnancy, a swift and blissful nine months, ended in unimaginable heartbreak when my baby daughter, Sierra, died just before she was born. My second pregnancy, an anxious eternity of medical tests and fretful nights, ended in the safe and happy delivery of my son, Skye. Despite their radically different outcomes, both pregnancies plugged me in to a connection with life—in all its beauty and mystery and terror—that was deeper and more powerful than I had ever dreamed possible.

If you're reading this book, you're probably pregnant or planning to be. And if you're anything like me, you probably have a thousand dreams and nightmares, conscious and unconscious, about your pregnancy, labor, and delivery: You will glow with happiness and good health. You will be swollen and repugnant, like a tick. You will go about your daily life without missing a beat. You will curl up in bed with baby-naming books while your husband rubs your feet and brings you vanilla milk shakes. You will have a home birth, without drugs or medical interventions, with sandalwood incense burning and Ravi Shankar playing on your stereo. Or you will have a tidy, planned C-section and get back to work in time to meet that big deadline. You will be Isis, the goddess of fertility. You will be the Wicked Witch of the West.

But your actual experience, as it unfolds moment by moment, will inevitably be different from your daydreams about it. Pregnancy, labor, and delivery form a journey of transformation on every level—physical, emotional, and spiritual. Like any pilgrimage, it will be full of surprises.

Being pregnant connects us to the central mystery of life as we experience—in pulsing, twitching, kicking intensity—a new human being coming into existence inside our own belly. It stitches us into the quilt of creation, binding us tightly to the generations that have come before and those that will come after. What better way to understand that there is no separate self—the core teaching of a host of spiritual traditions—than to share our every breath with another human being? What better way to smash through the walls of our limited egos than to devote our whole body to helping create another person?

But like all of life's great passages—birth, marriage, sex, death—pregnancy is not only extraordinary but also incredibly ordinary. Millions of women get pregnant every year; all of us were once cradled inside a woman's belly. The "miracle of pregnancy" is made up of a thousand mundane details: Your pants get tight. You puke at the sight of a burrito commercial. You own a dramatically increasing number of items with images of teddy bears on them.

You may not feel particularly saintly; in fact, you may be bored, nauseated, irritated, depressed. And when people try to tell you how miraculous this experience is—on a day when your hair is limp, your face is pimply, your breasts are sore, your butt won't fit into your maternity jeans, a weird brown stripe has descended from your belly button to your pubic hair, sciatica is shooting through your right hip, you've spent all night trying to find a comfortable sleeping position, and then every time you dozed off you had to get up and waddle to the bathroom to pee—you may be tempted to slap their faces.

As your sense of your own identity changes along with your underwear size, fears you'd like to dismiss as trivial can loom large: The thought that you'll no longer have the freedom to go to a rave on a Saturday night or a meditation retreat on a Sunday morning. The fear that you'll be nothing like your mother. The fear that you'll be exactly like your mother. The shock of not attracting a single lustful look as you waddle to the pool with your bikini tucked underneath your belly. The sudden conviction, at two A.M., that what you really wanted out of life was to go to Nepal and become a Buddhist nun.

Sometimes such anxieties mask other, more serious concerns. In the modern, Western world, pregnancy is overwhelmingly likely to culminate in a safe and healthy delivery. But the fact remains that any pregnancy puts us in touch with human frailty and vulnerability. We are never more aware of the preciousness of life than during pregnancy; we are also never more aware of its precariousness. In order to truly honor the miracle of our pregnancy, we must open our hearts to the possibility of devastating loss and disappointment.

Even the smoothest pregnancies have their moments of anxiety. There's the day when you don't feel your baby kick for hours. The decisions about whether to do tests such as amniocentesis, and the dark imaginings as you wait for the results. The passionate hopes for a boy or a girl—and the realization that you can't control who your baby is. The worries about the cocktail you had before you knew you were pregnant or the fumes from the new carpet being installed at your office or the blue cheese on your spinach salad.

The challenge, when such fears arise, is to face our vulnerability without contracting in terror. Our anxieties offer us the chance to drop straight into our hearts; to feel the tremendous love for our unborn child that underlies the worries; and to know that no matter what the outcome of our pregnancy, this love is itself a gift and a blessing.

I do have friends who have sailed through their pregnancies and deliveries without a hitch, everything going according to the blueprints of the *What to Expect* books. Many pregnancies have a magic sparkle about them, with everything falling into place with a mysterious synchronicity. My friend Adrianne's baby, Gracie, popped out on Christmas Eve, with big sister, Amelia, standing by to cut the cord. After a glowingly happy pregnancy, my friend Joanna's labor went so quickly and easily that her midwife didn't have time to get there, so Joanna and her husband delivered the baby on their own in their little backwoods cabin in Vermont.

But for many women, the story is more complicated. One

friend of mine, a massage therapist, labored for a day and a half in her candlelit bedroom before going to the hospital for an emergency C-section. Another friend's boyfriend bailed out the week after the home pregnancy test came up positive. My favorite yoga teacher spent her first trimester flat on her back in a darkened room, an IV in her arm, so nauseated that even water made her gag. My college roommate, who conceived in vitro, was on bed rest for the last two months of her pregnancy with triplets. My sister-in-law was on bed rest for most of her pregnancy because amniotic fluid kept leaking after her amniocentesis.

It's tempting to assume, when such storms rampage through our minds and bodies, that something has gone terribly wrong: that our pregnancy is no longer a spiritual journey. In our quest for the perfect natural childbirth, we may come to think the path of transformation is lit by candles, not by surgical lights, and that spiritual practice is somehow incompatible with medical technology. Most painful of all, we may believe that our most crushing losses represent a personal failure, thus piling self-judgment on top of heartbreak.

Ultimately, what makes pregnancy a spiritual practice is not what kind of pregnancy we have. It's how we open to it, moment by moment, breath by breath. Pregnancy is not about escaping or transcending physical existence. It's about embracing it, in all its grit and mess and blood and uncertainty and pain. Pregnancy pulls us straight into the heart of what it means to be alive. It reminds us we are part of a universe that is infinitely creative and breathtakingly beautiful but where, ultimately, most of what really matters is out of our personal control. It teaches us that life is both precious and fragile—and that our hearts are both bigger and more vulnerable than we could have imagined.

We often think of pregnancy as a time of waiting, a preamble to the real event of labor and delivery. Pregnant women are said to be "expectant" mothers, as if pregnancy is a waiting room where we peer out the window, counting the minutes until our baby's train arrives. But in reality, pregnancy is good in itself, a time when our child is cradled within us in a kind of intimacy we will never share again. Pregnancy invites us to cherish every moment of our baby's passage through us, knowing that, like life itself, it may end at any moment. In the midst of the gut-wrenching pain and grief when my first child was stillborn, my only comfort was the fact that I hadn't waited until she was born to love her, that I had treasured her for the whole nine months she lived inside me.

On the most basic, biological level, our consciousness is entwined with that of our unborn child. Our baby swims in a soup made partly of our hormones. He feels every beat of our heart, every surge of adrenaline, every milk shake and tofu scramble, every orgasm, every shudder. We can talk to her, dream about her, send her love, feel each tiny hiccup and kick of her legs.

The communication can have an eerie power. When I was thirty-nine weeks pregnant with my son, Skye, I was terrified that he, too, would die before being born, as Sierra had done at exactly that point in the pregnancy. My doctors offered me the option of easing my mind by inducing labor. Instead, my husband and I spoke with Skye, telling him how much we loved him, that the nest was all prepared, and that if he was ready, we would love to meet him as soon as possible. Perhaps it was a coincidence, but less than an hour after that ritual, my water broke and my contractions began.

If a meditative cherishing of every moment can turn pregnancy into a spiritual practice, it's also, I believe, what best prepares us for the drama of labor and delivery, the rite of passage that marks the final transition into motherhood. I think it's no accident that in tribal cultures around the world, it's men who feel the need for painful and bloody rituals that mark the transition from child to adult. Women have never needed to create such rituals. We have one built into our own life cycle. Labor and delivery call upon strength and courage and willpower we didn't know we had while simultaneously demanding that we surrender to a process that is fundamentally out of our control. They split us open, turn us inside out, yank off our masks of self-control and ego.

We generally think of spiritual practice as something tidy as a temple, smelling of jasmine and sandalwood. But for most of us, labor and delivery are wild and messy and animal and angry and bloody and painful. The transcendent act of giving birth is made up of the earthiest of elements: bodily fluids, a hospital gown stained with blood and excrement, the bruises left on your partner's arm by the agonized grip of your fingers.

You may find yourself howling like a cat, throwing up on the rug, emptying your bowels on the sheets of your bed, hurling curses at your beloved husband or dearest friend. You may get up off the delivery table in the middle of labor—like my friend Linda—and announce to the doctors that you're going home, that you've changed your mind and aren't going to have a baby after all.

Midway through my own labor with my son, Skye, things seemed to have stalled. I had stopped at six centimeters of dilation; the contractions were continuing but not increasing in intensity. "You're afraid of feeling more pain," said my midwife, Angelika, who blends compassion with a samurai's ferocity when necessary. "So you're stopping the labor. You want the baby to be born, but you don't want the pain to get any worse. But in order for the baby to be born, the pain will have to increase. You will have to go past what you think is your limit."

I had been a student of yoga and meditation for almost twenty years by then. I had chosen natural childbirth because I wanted to feel every moment of my child coming into the world, wanted his mind and my mind unclouded by drugs as we looked into each other's eyes for the first time. I was strongly attached to being in control of my experience, and I thought there was no pain I couldn't breathe into. Yet, as I opened to the pain of childbirth, there I was cursing, thrashing, growling like an animal, hitting the side of my hospital bed. "Goddamn it," I screamed. "Get me the fucking epidural!"

But by then, of course, it was too late for the epidural. The urge blazed through me, a wave, a convulsion, my whole body clamping down in an involuntary push. A ring of fire seemed to be opening between my legs. Next to me, my husband was beside himself with excitement—"Here he is, he's almost here"—but in that moment, I didn't even care that I was having a baby. I just wanted the pain to go away.

Someone put my hand down to feel my baby's head. "Let it in," I thought. "Let it out."

And then there was a heave and a great release, and a baby was crying; and my hands were reaching down and pulling a slippery, slithery bundle onto my chest.

"Hello, Skye," said my husband, Lou. And Skye, only seconds old, lifted his wobbly head off my chest and turned it to look, with bleary, unfocused eyes, in the direction of his daddy's voice.

The memory of Skye's birth has become a talisman that I hold in my heart as I journey deeper and deeper into motherhood. For these moments come again and again in every mother's life—the times when we are asked to walk straight into our pain and fear, and in doing so, open up to a love that is greater than anything we ever could have imagined. Our hearts expand to embrace everything: all life's beauty and wonder, as well as all the ways that things can break and go wrong.

As mothers, we discover that we love our children in whatever form they are in: a kicking bulge in our womb, a baby sucking at our breast, a toddler leaving Play-Doh crumbs on the couch, a pierced and tattooed teenager blasting rap music at midnight. We love them when they're ill and when they are damaged. We love them long after they have died. And in discovering this, we open to a kind of love that transcends form and time. It's at the heart of our humanness, yet you might call it divine.

Again and again, motherhood demands that we break through our limitations, that we split our hearts open to make room for something that may be more than we thought we could bear. In that sense, the labor with which we give birth is simply a rehearsal for something we mothers must do over and over: turn ourselves inside out, and then let go.

PRACTICE

Basic Breath Awareness

CD TRACK 3

The best tool we have for working with the ebb and flow of our feelings and experiences is always with us: our own breath. Regular breathwork during pregnancy can be a wonderful preparation for childbirth. This can be as simple as counting out ten slow, deep breaths, making sure the inhalation and exhalation are of equal length. Or you can set aside some time each day of your pregnancy to breathe, meditate, and allow yourself to relax into this experience. Here's one way to do so:

1. Find a quiet, comfortable place to sit. You can sit on a chair with both feet resting on the ground or on a cushion with crossed legs. Sit up straight and relaxed with both hands resting on your thighs. If you are tense or perching, let yourself settle. If you tend to slouch, sit up. Notice how it feels to be physically still. Notice the movement within stillness.

2. Take a few moments to settle in, and then gradually begin paying attention to your breath. It's helpful to

focus your attention either at the tip of the nose or at the abdomen. There's no need to control or change your breathing; simply notice the sensation of breathing in and breathing out. Let your mind ride the cycle of the breath.

3. When you notice that your attention has moved off the breath and is now absorbed in thought or sensation, simply bring your mind back to your breath. No matter how thrilling, terrifying, boring, or irritating your thoughts may have been, just let them dissolve and come back to the breath. Just keep coming back.

Sitting this way for even ten minutes a day can bring enormous benefit.

> *Pregnancy is a chance for awakening. If spiritual masters counsel us to put others before ourselves, be in the present moment, understand that we are not separate from each other, and live in awe of all living things—what brings us to these awarenesses better than carrying a baby?*
>
> —Michelle

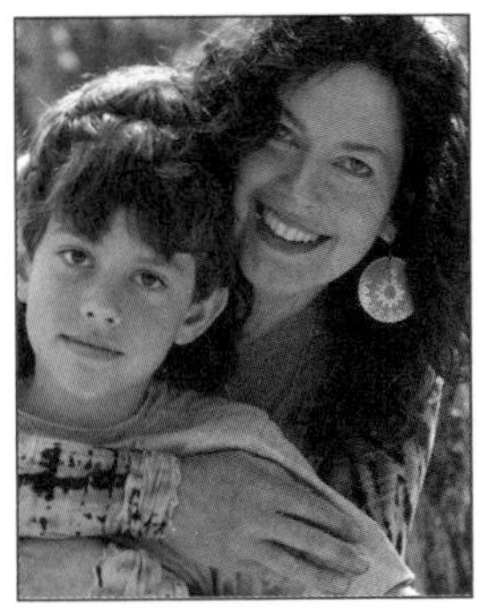

About

Anne Cushman

As a writer and teacher of yoga and Buddhist meditation, Anne Cushman has been investigating the relationship between Eastern spiritual traditions and contemporary Western life for more than twenty-five years.

Anne is a longtime contributor and former editor at both *Yoga Journal* and *Tricycle: The Buddhist Review*. Her personal essays have also appeared in the *New York Times*, the *San Francisco Chronicle*, *O: The Oprah Magazine*, Salon.com, *New Woman*, and the *Shambhala Sun*. Her work has been anthologized in *Best Buddhist Writing 2004* and *2006; Best Women's Spiritual Travel Writing; Traveling Souls: Contemporary Pilgrimage Tales;* and other books.

She has practiced Buddhist meditation since 1983 in both the Zen and Vipassana traditions, and is the codirector of the Mindfulness Yoga and Meditation Training Program at Spirit Rock Meditation Center in Woodacre, California.

She lives in Fairfax, California, with her ten-year-old son, Skye Hawthorne.

When we practice yoga to nurture ourselves, we are also nurturing the babies who are growing in us.

2

Nurturing Your Body with Yoga

Jennifer Brilliant

Yoga is a powerful practice for living: It engages us physically, intellectually, emotionally, and spiritually. It helps us live well. As we move our bodies, we begin to understand more about ourselves and the world around us. Our feelings, which reside in our muscles, bones, and nerves, are unearthed and resettled. Because it increases our awareness, yoga is not only a physical practice but also a spiritual one. It is especially helpful when we are pregnant and our bodies are changing rapidly in ways that may seem disorienting. Pregnancy is a major life passage, and yoga keeps us attuned to the process. It also offers us something tangible to do with our stress, doubt, and fear. Thus, it can alleviate and even prevent not only physical but emotional discomforts that may accompany pregnancy.

When we practice yoga to nurture ourselves, we are also nurturing the babies who are growing in us. Yoga postures help keep our arms and legs strong and supple so that we can support the extra weight we carry during pregnancy. This, in turn, allows us to offer our babies a stable and healthy environment to swim around in while they are developing.

Since the time I was a little girl, I had the idea that being pregnant would make me feel ungainly and awful. Luckily, I was completely wrong. I practiced and taught yoga throughout my forty-one weeks of carrying my daughter, Mollie. Of course, during my pregnancy, my yoga practice changed a lot. But even though I modified some of the postures I normally practice, and omitted others altogether, I still felt many benefits. My pregnancy (at age forty-one) was a magical and wonderful time. Teaching yoga nearly every day required that I embrace the changes in my body, a process that felt absolutely natural and required little effort on my part. I found that if I just showed up in yoga class, whether as teacher or as student, I left with a quieter nervous system and a calmer mind.

I suggest you take the time to practice yoga at home, even

if it is just for a few minutes a day. Choose a place with enough room for a yoga mat. (The mat helps prevent you from slipping while you're doing the poses.) To begin, sit quietly and observe your breath for a few moments to find your own natural rhythm. You can practice the poses in the sequence in which they're listed here or in any other order, or you can do only the poses that interest you. It's totally okay to rest between poses; this way, you have the possibility of digesting the effects of each pose.

I suggest variations on some of the poses. The variations are done with props: blankets, blocks, or a belt. Using these props can improve your alignment, which affects your body's energy flow. By using blankets or other props, you can always find a way to get the benefits of any pose.

The instructions I offer here include important tips for pregnant women practicing yoga. Please read the instructions carefully and always consult your doctor if you have any questions or concerns.

General Guidelines for Yoga during Pregnancy

- Stay in each pose for as long as you can focus well on your breath and as long as the pose feels beneficial for you.

- Listen to your body. If you listen attentively, it will tell you what to do. If a pose doesn't feel good, back out of it a bit and breathe—or back out of it altogether.

- You don't have to do every pose. Choose the ones that feel right for you.

- Be disciplined with your practice, but be willing to adjust based on how you feel each day.

- There are special constraints on yoga practice during the first three months of pregnancy, especially if you have had a miscarriage in the past. As with every form of physical exercise, it's best to get personal advice from your doctor or an experienced teacher.

- Yoga postures should be adapted to maintain a respectful space for your belly. Avoid deep forward bending, which can cramp baby's style.

- Avoid twists, too; they also compress the abdomen, and the action of twisting mimics the movement of uterine contractions. We don't want to contract until we have carried the baby to full term!

- Backbends are fine for some pregnant women and not for others. Backbends can exacerbate *diastasis recti,* a separation of the abdominal muscles that some women develop during pregnancy. If you have any doubt about whether you can do backbends safely, check with your doctor. It's best to be cautious.

May you and your baby be happy and safe, and may you live with ease and peace.

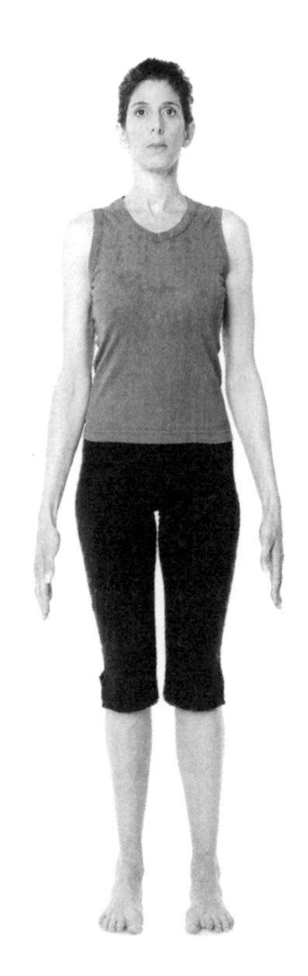

MOUNTAIN POSE

Stand with your feet about hip-distance apart. Spread your feet so that the balls of your feet feel wide and supportive. Feel your weight balanced on the front of your heel bone. A quality of broadness in your feet can help you to feel grounded. Engage your leg muscles to create strong and active legs. Balance the center of your pelvis directly over the front of your heel bones. Be aware of the natural curve of your lower back. The pull of the belly forward can cause the lower back to overarch, or you may be compensating by tucking your tail under. Think long and strong in your low back. Lift your rib cage with buoyancy above your pelvis. Let the summit of your mountain (your shoulders and head) enjoy the view of yourself as a soon-to-be mom.

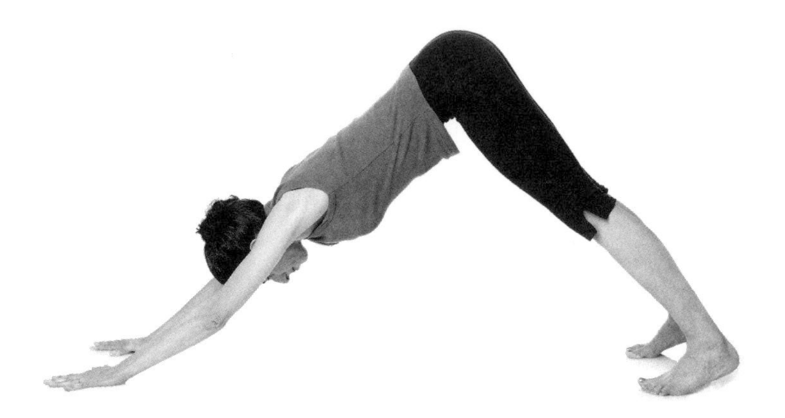

DOWNWARD-FACING DOG

This pose strengthens and stretches the arms and legs while opening the spine. Begin on all fours. Release your hands down and strongly lift your wrist bones up. This helps to keep space in the wrist joint and will lessen any compression there. Tuck your toes under and lift both knees simultaneously off the floor. To straighten your legs, lift your sitting bones upward, which opens your hamstrings, and release your heels downward (they may not reach the floor), which opens your calves. Move the weight of your body back toward your legs. This pose reverses the relationship of your womb to gravity. So, if your baby is in the head-down position, she now has her head upright. Thus, this pose gives both you and your little one a new perspective. To release, bend your knees simultaneously and place them back on the floor in the beginning position.

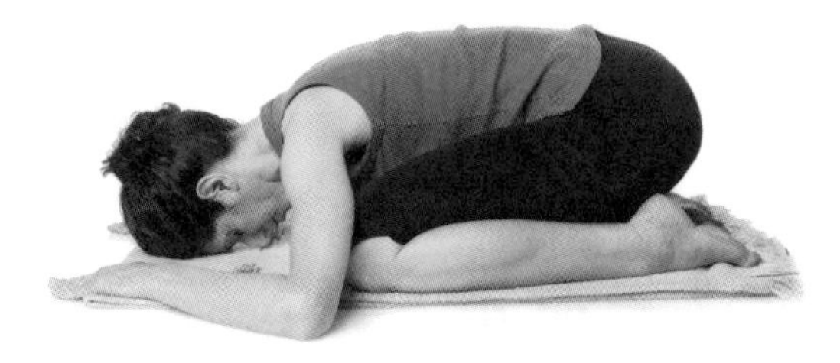

CHILD'S POSE

For physical, mental, and emotional balance it is beneficial to spend time relaxing. Child's Pose can release tension in the lower back. It is also a good way to feel your breath. Begin on all fours with your knees wider than your hips but with your feet toward each other. (This variation with the knees wide will accommodate your belly during your pregnancy.) Sit your buttocks back onto your heels. If there is any discomfort in your knees, place some padding between your feet and your buttocks. Rest your forehead on the floor or on your hands. If your head doesn't release down to your hands, place your head on a block. Child's Pose gives you an opportunity to nurture yourself like a little embryo. Let yourself be the baby, soft and fluid.

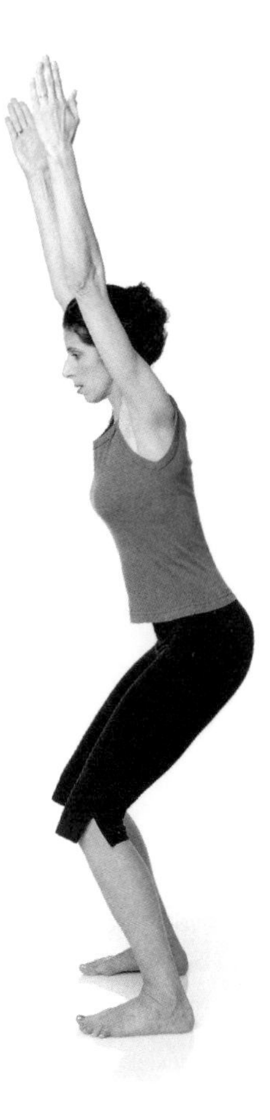

CHAIR POSE

This challenging pose can give a feeling of power in your legs. With your feet hip-distance apart, bend your knees and sit back with your pelvis. Keep your chest lifted and your back open. Raise your arms up alongside your ears with your hands as wide as your shoulders, or rest your hands on your thighs. As you deepen into this pose, you will feel your thigh muscles. See if you can also feel a stretch in your lower calves. You may have to sit back farther to feel this. Work to lift the arches of your feet so that they maintain their support.

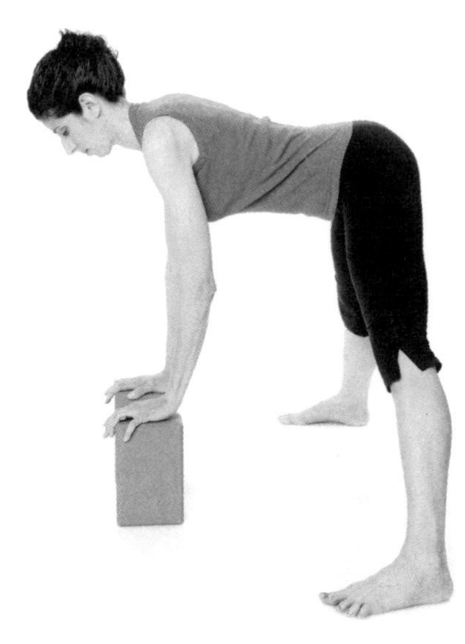

SPREAD-LEG FORWARD BEND

This pose will stretch your hamstrings and inner thighs while leaving optimal space for your baby, your breath, and all of your internal organs. It is also a good way to strengthen your legs and ankles. Stand with your legs in a wide parallel position. Place your hands on your waist. Folding at your hip crease, bend forward, keeping your spine long. Place your hands on blocks or on the seat of a chair as wide as your shoulders. Feel your hands and feet reaching down to Mother Earth as you lengthen up at the very tops of your thighs.

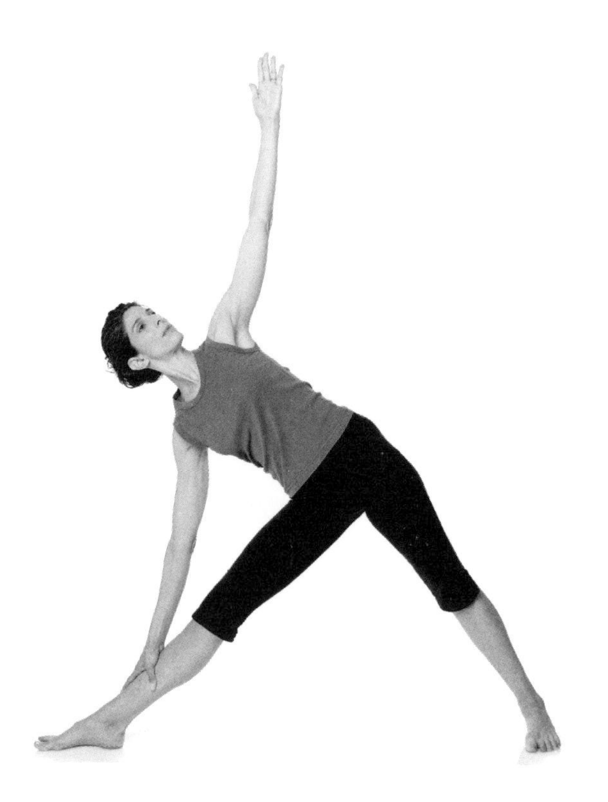

TRIANGLE POSE

Stand with your feet parallel and wide apart. Turn your left foot inward slightly. Then turn your right foot ninety degrees to your right. Spread your arms open at shoulder level. Bend laterally as you move to the right. Press your right hand on your right shin or place your fingertips to the outside of your right foot on the floor. Your left arm reaches upward toward the sky. Turn your face upward in coordination with your chest lifting. This pose is a practical and tangible way to work on balance. Find the balance between a trusting release into gravity and a directed rebound away from it. To come out of the pose, turn your right foot inward so that you are in the wide parallel stance. Either immediately repeat on the left side or bend your knees to step your feet together for Mountain Pose, to rest before continuing.

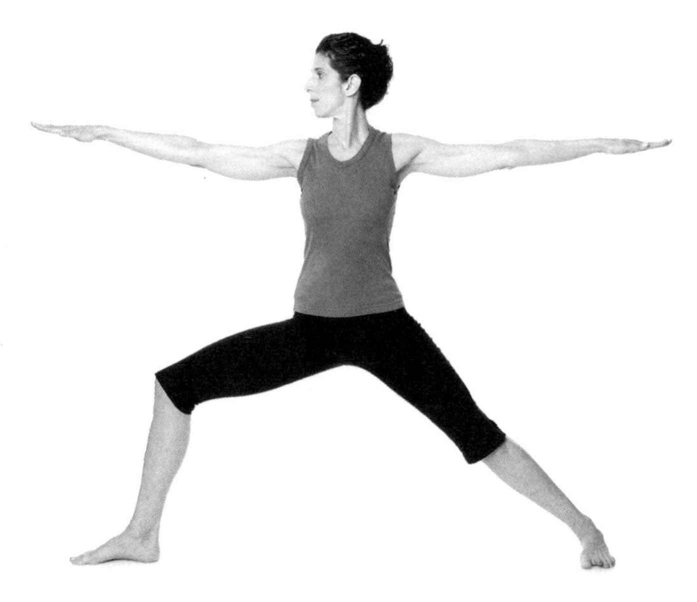

WARRIOR II

The openness and strength of Warrior II are a metaphor for our self-reliance. From Mountain Pose, open your legs into a wide parallel position. Turn your left foot inward slightly and your right foot out ninety degrees. Bend your right knee as you lift your arms up to shoulder level with the palms facing down. The gaze extends out beyond your right hand. Keep your right thigh and knee facing directly over but not beyond your right foot. To release, come back to a vertical stance by straightening your right leg with your arms open at shoulder level. Place your hands on your waist. Turn your right foot inward so that you are back in the wide parallel stance. Repeat on the left side, or else bend your knees to step your feet together for Mountain Pose and rest before continuing.

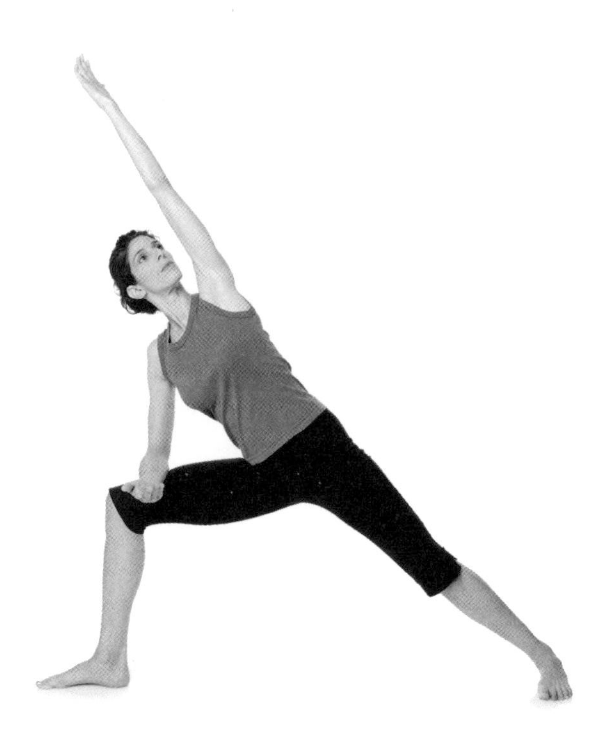

EXTENDED SIDE-ANGLE POSE

This pose opens the chest, hips, and spine. Begin in a wide stance with feet parallel. Turn your left foot inward. Turn your right foot ninety degrees toward the right. Lift your arms to shoulder level. Keeping your right buttock underneath you, bend your right knee. Place your right forearm on your right thigh. It is okay to lean on the forearm because your right leg offers good support. Move your left arm up alongside your left ear. If possible, revolve so that you can gaze upward. If you feel strain in your neck, you can look straight ahead or down. To release, come to a vertical stance by straightening your right leg with your arms open at shoulder level. Turn your right foot inward so that you are back in parallel stance. Repeat on the left side, or else place your hands on your waist, bend your knees to step your feet together for Mountain Pose, and rest before continuing.

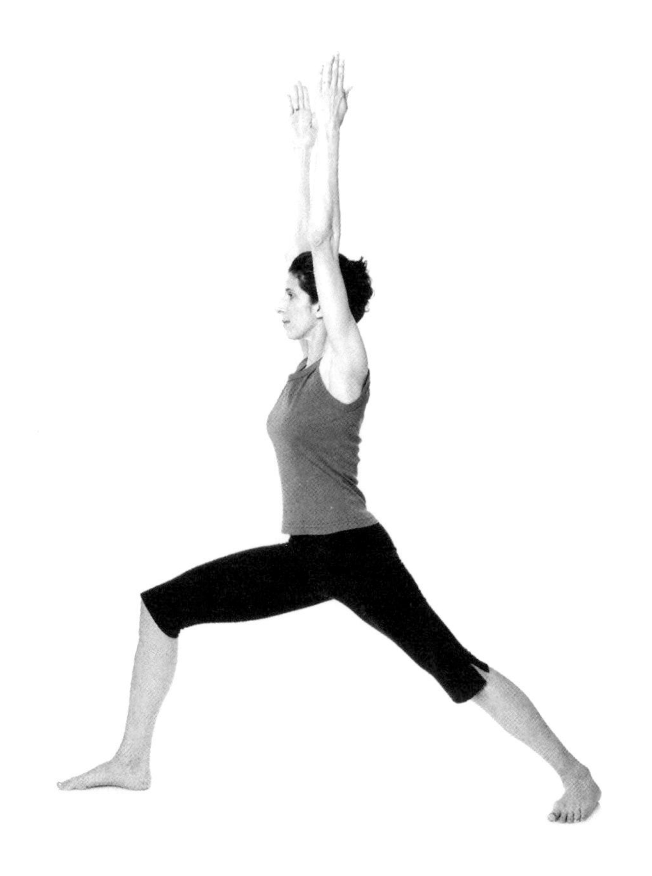

WARRIOR I

Open your legs to a wide parallel position. Turn your left foot in about sixty degrees. Bend your front knee. Reach your left heel down into the earth as best you can. Raise your arms up, palms facing each other. Your nose, chest, and knee all face fearlessly forward. You can practice Warrior I with your hands on your waist to reduce fatigue. (If you have high blood pressure, keep your hands on your waist in any case.) Stay present with your breath and body to develop stamina, strength, and bravery. Practicing Warrior I will train you to use these qualities skillfully when you are faced with challenges, such as giving birth. To release, straighten your right leg. Turn your right foot so you are back in the wide parallel stance, hands on waist. Repeat on the left side, or else bend your knees to step your feet together for Mountain Pose and rest before continuing.

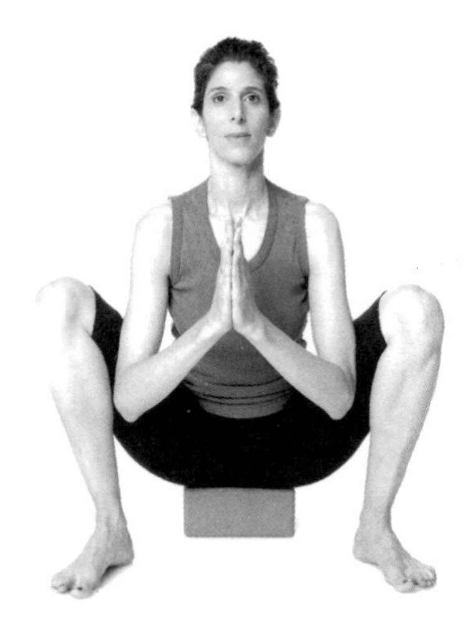

SQUAT POSE

Squatting can soften and broaden the pelvic floor, which can help the baby to descend. Opening your hips in a squat can also help relieve tension in your back. Stand with your feet wider than your hips. Bend your knees and lower down to sit on a block. Keep your chest lifted. Bring your elbows to the inside of your knees, and place your palms against each other in Prayer Pose. Your block can be placed at any height. You want to feel some opening, but it shouldn't be uncomfortable. To release, stretch both legs out simultaneously in a way that feels good to you.

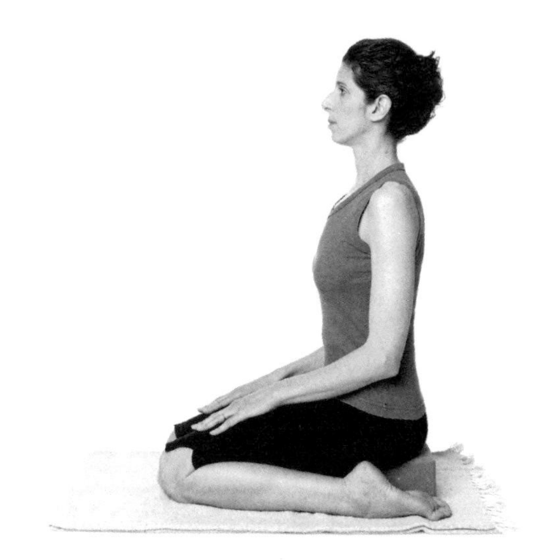

HERO'S POSE

Begin on all fours, with knees together and feet separated enough so that you can sit back on a block that is between your feet. Your feet are lined up just outside your thighbones, toes facing back. Rest your hands on your thighs. If you experience any difficulty in your knees, raise your buttocks higher using another block or a blanket. If that still doesn't help, place a folded washcloth into the back of your knee creases as you sit down. If your feet or ankles are uncomfortable, put some padding under the tops of your feet or under your ankles. Hero's Pose is therapeutic for the hips, knees, and feet. To exit this pose like a hero, tuck your toes under and lift into Downward-Facing Dog. Let your sitting bones and hamstrings lift up, but release your heels and calves down, allowing your knees to align smoothly with your legs.

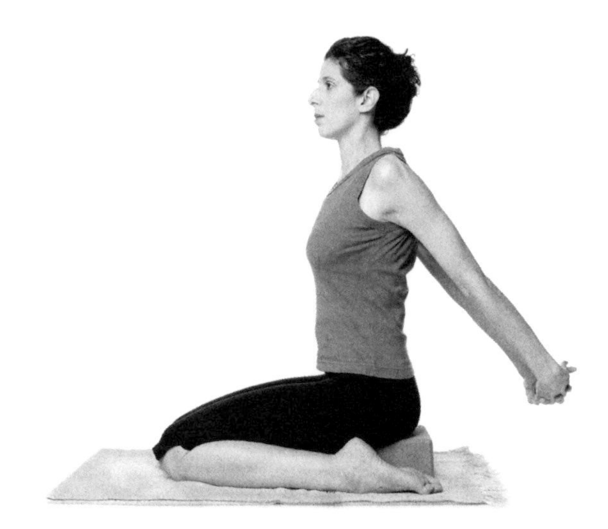

HERO'S POSE: CHEST-OPENING VARIATION

Opening your shoulders and chest will help you keep a dignified posture as you nurse and nurture your little one. Interlace your fingers behind your back and move your hands back and up away from you. If your hands don't come together yet, grasping a belt with both hands can help.

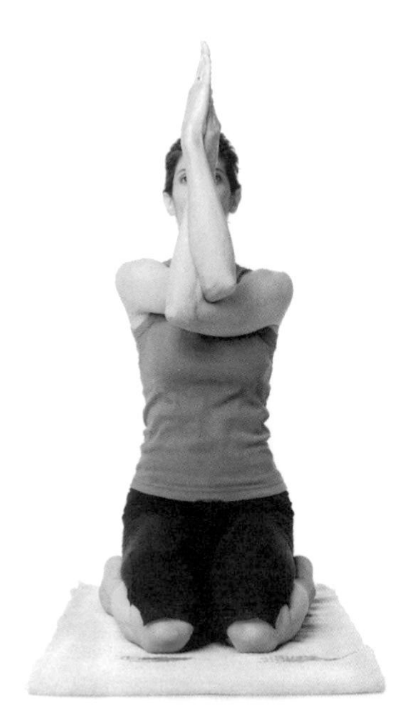

EAGLE ARMS

In this variation of Hero's Pose, you can feel the spread at the back of the shoulders and in the upper back. Extend your arms out to your sides at shoulder level. Cross your straight arms above the elbows in front of your chest, north of your breasts. First the right elbow crosses above the left elbow. Then bend your arms, snuggling your elbows into each other so that your forearms stretch upward with your thumbs facing toward your head. To intertwine your hands around each other, move your left hand toward your face and your right hand away from you. Cross your hands bringing your palms together. Raise your elbows up to the level of your shoulders. Release by stretching your arms out to your sides at shoulder level. Repeat with the left arm on top.

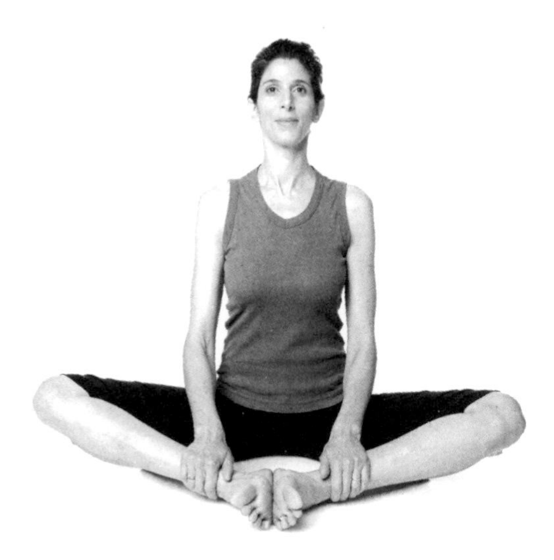

BOUND ANGLE POSE

This pose is practice for opening up your pelvis during childbirth. Sit on the floor or on a folded blanket. This helps maintain alignment of pelvis and spine. Bend your knees, open them, and place the soles of your feet together. Place your hands on your ankles. Create an energetic movement of your thighs away from your pubic bone toward your knees. Let your pubic bone reach down toward the floor. This will give you a feeling of openness in the low belly and your pelvic floor. You can easily feel a stretch in the hips and inner thighs. Be willing to go more deeply and open at your very base. By letting your breath move into your pelvic floor, you create a wavelike motion that will give Junior a very gentle massage. On the inhalation, feel your pelvic floor open, and on the exhale, draw your pelvic floor muscles up.

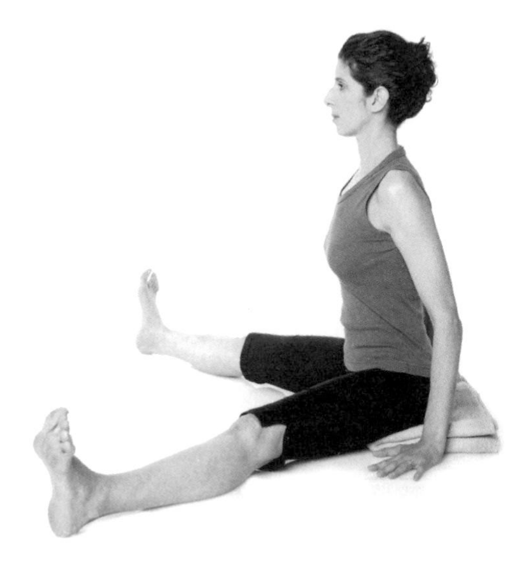

OPEN ANGLE POSE

Sit on the floor or on a folded blanket. Open your legs into a wide straddle. Flex your feet so that your heels reach away from you. Your legs are in good alignment when your knees and your toes face up toward the sky. Opening the hips and legs like this will bring vitality to your pelvic region. Reach toward your feet with yogic toe lock, wrapping your second and third fingers between your big toe and second toe, or hold on to your shins. If you are flexible, narrow your legs so that you can reach your feet for yogic toe lock. If you are tight in the hips, this pose can increase your flexibility. If you are already flexible, this pose will help develop strength and a feeling of grounded support.

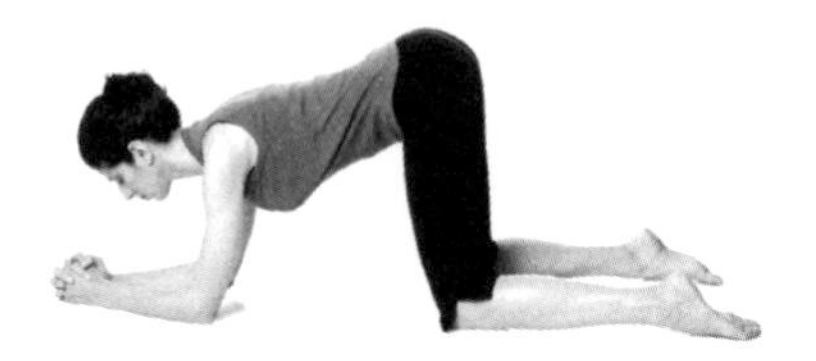

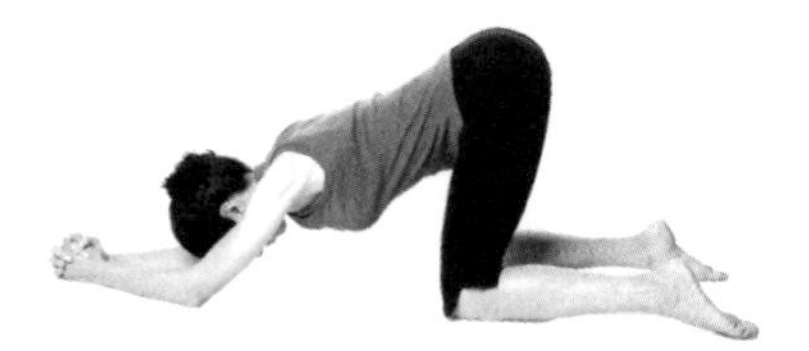

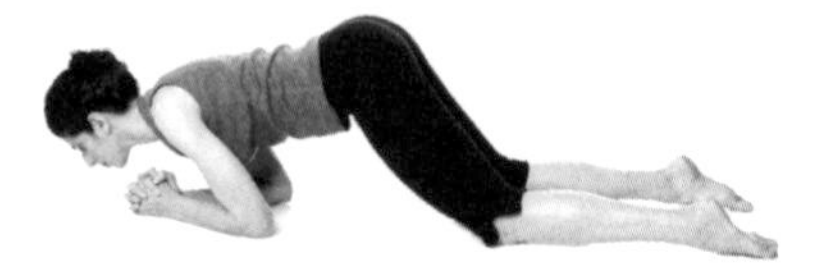

DOLPHIN POSE

Even before birth, our developing baby demands our energy and attention. This pose helps to keep our bodies energetically balanced by increasing the feeling of vitality and lift in the upper body. Start on all fours, then lower your elbows to the floor, one at a time, directly under your shoulders. Interlace your fingers so that you create a tripod between your hands and your two elbows. Press your elbows, forearms, wrists, and the outer edge of your hands into the floor to create a strong foundation.

Move your chest back toward your thighs, keeping your arms grounded.

Then shift your weight forward until your face comes above or even past your hands.

You can repeat this several times to feel the muscles that connect your rib cage to your shoulders and arms.

Move back to the start position. Repeat several times.

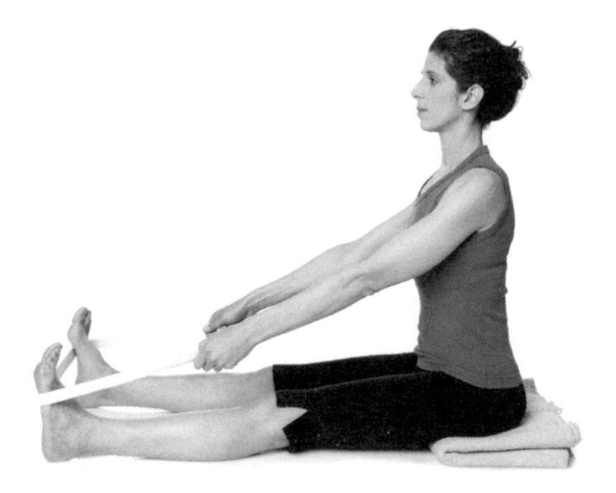

SEATED FORWARD BEND

This pose can be calming. Sit on the floor, legs outstretched and wider than your hips, so that your belly has complete freedom. If you feel strain in your back, sit on a folded blanket. Activate your leg muscles and feet. Your legs are aligned when knees and toes face directly up to the ceiling. Rotate your legs a bit to find this alignment. The feet are flexed, but the heels do not leave the floor. Imagine that your sitting bones and your heels can move away from each other, creating more space in the hip crease. Move into this space as you reach your arms forward with an open chest to hold your shins, ankles, feet, or a belt wrapped around your feet. Extend your back long and wide. During labor, the release of the thighs downward can give relief during contractions. My husband helped me during labor by leaning his weight down on my thighs in this and other positions.

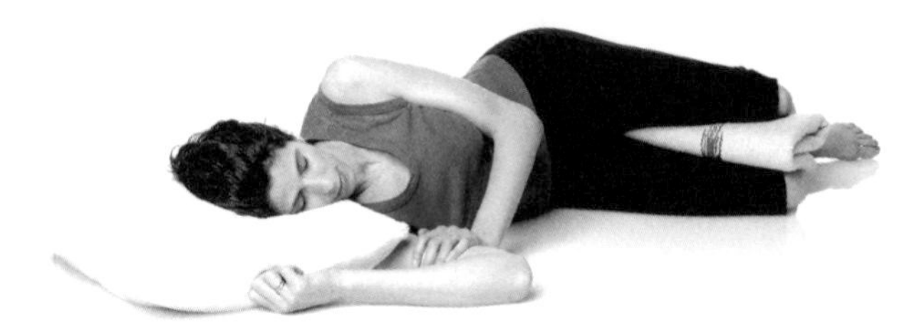

CORPSE POSE

Practicing being relaxed will help you to live with more relaxation. During pregnancy some women feel uncomfortable lying on their backs; others feel okay in that position. Each pregnant woman is unique and should be guided by her own comfort. If you decide to lie on your back, your legs can be slightly open and your arms far enough away from your sides so that your breath feels free. The palms face up and have a very soft quality so that your fingers curl naturally. This is a gesture of offering. Offer yourself to this time of relaxation. If you decide to lie on your side, place a pillow between your knees and one under your head. Use this time to rest or have a quiet talk with your baby.

PRACTICE

Aromatherapy for Pregnancy

Essential oils can soothe, stimulate, and balance physical and emotional energies.

Because they're very potent, never apply essential oils directly to the body; always mix them with "carrier" oils. Any vegetable oil will serve as a carrier oil, but Daphne Seligmann Hagadone, owner of Daphne Studio in New York City, which specializes in using essential oils as part of its spa treatments, recommends apricot, almond, coconut, hazelnut, and olive oils. The rule of thumb is to mix two to three drops of essential oil per tablespoon of carrier oil, with one exception: rose oil. Rose oil is so potent that Daphne suggests using only one to two drops per tablespoon of carrier oil.

- Use rose oil on your face to soothe rashes and lessen discoloration. Rose oil can also stabilize mood; it is said to strengthen the heart and release fear.
- Rub mandarin or rose oils on your belly to prevent stretch marks. During her pregnancy, Daphne used both

oils twice a day and gives these treatments the credit for her stretch mark–free belly.

- Mandarin oil also can lift depression and elevate mood.
- Applied to the belly or simply smelled, jasmine oil promotes relaxation and can help ease nausea and even the pain of early labor.
- Lavender oil also relaxes the nervous system.

Remember

Always dilute the essential oils in a carrier oil. Experiment with combinations that smell and feel good to your body.

Note

Aromatherapists advise against applying oils to the scalp or feet during pregnancy; these can overstimulate the reproductive organs.

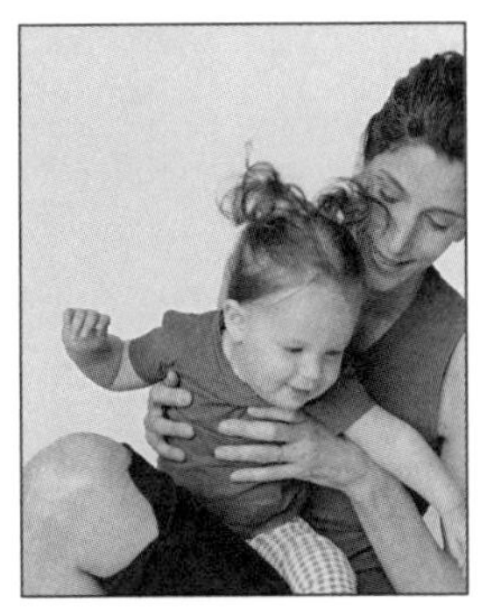

About

Jennifer Brilliant

Jennifer Brilliant has twenty-five years of experience guiding people in athletic, therapeutic, and creative movement. Her vast knowledge of the human body is drawn from the Pilates method, the Alexander Technique, Kinetic Awareness, meditation instruction in the Shambhala tradition, and ten years as a professional modern dancer with Jennifer Muller / The Works. Since 1989 Jennifer has taught one-on-one fitness and yoga in homes and offices throughout New York City. Her company, Jennifer Brilliant Yoga and Personal Training, offers movement education and training.

Jennifer teaches all levels of group and private yoga classes in New York City and leads special workshops across the country. She was the director of the OM yoga center's teacher training programs from 2000 to 2005. Under her careful eye, dozens of graduates have become OM-certified yoga teachers.

We will connect and separate, connect and separate for the rest of our lives.

3

Bonding with Your Baby

Celia Straus

The formation of our unborn child goes hand in hand with the formation of the most intimate human relationship possible. Begun at conception, this bonding process continues all through our lives, but for the first few months it is unfamiliar territory. Although brief, this phase of the mother-child relationship brings with it a complex range of emotions, from overwhelming love and joyful anticipation to fear, frustration, and resentment—all of which I experienced during pregnancy with my second daughter.

Five months into this risky pregnancy, I was advised to go to bed and stay there. By putting my life on pause, I discovered that the emotional bonds between my inner self and this new fledgling self were as real as the physical ones. Without speaking aloud, I carried on continuous one-way conversations with my daughter, encouraging her to grow and thrive. We were partners, teammates working together on a heart or lung development project. When I ate a meal, I mentally asked her how she liked it. When I heard a song I particularly liked, I promised her we'd go hear the group in concert, together. My inner voice whispered to her throughout our days and nights. Although I can never be sure intellectually that she heard these inner monologues, in my heart I believe she did.

Yet by making the bonding process my personal project, I put myself through needless worry. When I didn't feel my daughter move, I became fearful. When I wanted to scream out of boredom or out of resentment at being told to sleep on my left side only (which is virtually impossible to sustain once you're asleep, assuming you can sleep), I was overcome with guilt. Since at times I had to become vertical as the temporarily disengaged but still working mother of a four-year-old, I was often ambivalent, concerned that whatever choice I made was the wrong one. When I thought about how much I wanted this baby, I was awed by the intensity of my feelings.

It took months of enforced solitude to learn how to surrender myself to the Divine, allowing it to grow and shape my daughter. But eventually I relaxed. I stopped trying to force myself to feel the emotions that I imagined would improve the bonding process and subtly promote a healthy birth. Only then, when I avoided thinking about feeling happiness, contentment, joyful anticipation, or anything maternal, did I feel a true connection between the two of us. Only when I gave up all attempts to control, judge, or program my emotions did I begin to trust this powerful bond, which was also as ephemeral as a gentle breeze.

If we can stop second-guessing ourselves and forcing ourselves to feel whatever we're conditioned to believe we ought to feel, bonding will simply happen. We wait, filled with awe at our capacity to create and to love our creation without ever having seen it. We wait, certain that the closer we come to birthing, the more our performance anxiety will grow, and the worse we will perform. Which mother hasn't been caught off guard by the mood swings and contradictory emotions that go along with pregnancy? In the course of one day we can go from feeling as if we were one with our unborn child and the universe to feeling resentment that our lives will never be the same, or frustration that our bodies—so distorted that we cannot see our own feet while standing—are no longer our own. And after we feel that, we also feel guilty for having felt anything negative.

We can, however, experience our pregnancy another way, by adding a spiritual dimension. Motherhood offers us one of the most direct opportunities we will ever have to experience our humanity more fully. We may even discover that bonding involves unconditional love that transcends whatever phase of life mother and child may be experiencing, from pregnancy on. We may learn not to hold ourselves responsible for being a "good" expectant mother or for successfully mothering our newborn. Instead, with open hearts, we can trust that the basic goodness and reliability of the Divine, in life and in ourselves, will care for our baby better than we ever could.

If we approach our impending motherhood this way, we are giving both ourselves and our child a great gift. We are building a strong yet flexible structure for a successful mother-child relationship, which, sure as the sunrise, will continue to change and evolve. We are creating bonds that will withstand the inevitable contradictions of motherhood: the positive and negative feelings about our child, the closeness of connection and pain of separation, the self-confidence we achieve as we get better at mothering and the despair when we fail at it. As our children grow older, for example, we can better meet the challenges of separation. Separation, of course, is seldom easy. It begins at birth, and from that miraculous moment on, we will connect and separate, connect and separate for the rest of our lives. But relaxing with the natural ebb and flow of feelings and connectedness gives us balance and perspective, and thus separation comes to seem as natural as any other part of our relationship.

Once, when I was working on a television series about shamans, I was also recovering from the emotional trauma of a miscarriage. In the midst of an interview with a very wise, very old Native American woman, I found myself pouring out my story. She patted my arm and told me not to worry. That little soul, she told me, had desired only a brief existence here on earth. Another child's soul would soon choose me, she promised, and this little girl-soul would insist that we, together, experience her birth. And, indeed, a year later, my second daughter was born. What I took away from my conversation with the old woman was that we should be quietly aware of the creation process within us and accept all we feel about our unborn child's living presence without judgment. Let us take these precious few months to learn better how to love ourself and our baby, unconditionally and with spirit.

PRACTICE

Tonglen Meditation

CD TRACK 5

Tonglen literally means "sending and taking," and in tonglen meditation, we practice sending out warmth and kindness to others and taking away their fear or pain. At the same time we examine our own fears and attachments, actually taking in what we fear and letting go of what we desire. By freeing us from our habits of fear and self-absorption, tonglen can lead us to greater acceptance and loving-kindness—both for ourselves and for others. It bonds us to all beings.

Like motherhood, tonglen is very basic. It has nothing to do with being a goody-goody or pretending to be nice when we really feel otherwise. Rather, it is based on acceptance. No matter what we're feeling—inspired or uninspired, nauseated or well, loving or resentful, beautiful or ugly, frightened or confident—in tonglen practice, we simply breathe in what we do not want and breathe out what we do.

For new mothers, tonglen can be extremely useful. It teaches us to work straightforwardly with difficulties and extend ourselves more wholeheartedly to others. It shows us more clearly how the extremes of loathing and attachment can rule us. We see, for instance, how the perfectionistic image of the self-sacrificing, all-accommodating mother can lead us to become its exact opposite: the resentful, suffocating mother. It shows us how damaging it is to fear and deny our feelings if they do not fit our image of what a good mother should be. In the practice of tonglen, we sit, if only briefly, and reverse this pattern. As we breathe in, we invite in all those messy feelings. As we breathe out, we let go of clinging to being right and good and perfect. The change is refreshing.

The practice of tonglen has four steps:

1. The first step is very brief. You can think of it as clearing the decks. Simply allow a little pause, or gap, before you begin your sending and taking. Although brief and simple, this step is still important. It's like cracking the window to let in a little fresh air.

2. In the second step you begin the process of sending and taking. Each time you breathe in, breathe in heavy, dark, claustrophobic energy; and each time you breathe out,

breathe out light, refreshing, clear, cool energy. With each breath, you will feel an ongoing rhythm, back and forth. You are reversing the habit of grasping and rejecting.

3. In the third step, you notice whatever arises in your mind and apply the tonglen practice to that. Work with a topic that arouses real feelings, something that actually touches you or feels a little raw. It doesn't need to be anything monumental; it can be quite ordinary. For instance, you can breathe in the feeling of being overwhelmed and tired and breathe out the feeling of being energetic. Or you can breathe in your fear that you will not make a good mother and breathe out your wish to be a supermom. The point is to start with something that has some reality or juice in your life.

4. In the fourth step you expand the practice beyond your own concerns. For instance, if you're worried about your baby's health, expand that concern to include all the other people now and in the past who have had similar worries. Breathe in all those worries and breathe out to all those countless beings your wish that they be freed from such pain. In this way you link your journey to the journeys of mothers before and after you, near and far away.

The Zen teaching "Only don't know" is a great motto for the journey of pregnancy and motherhood. There's so much uncertainty and vulnerability, and our fears can easily push us to the edge. "Only don't know" reminds me to allow the uncertainty to be there. It reminds me not to rush in with my expectations and preconceptions, to remain open to whatever shows up. Sitting meditation gives me practice in doing that.

—Eden

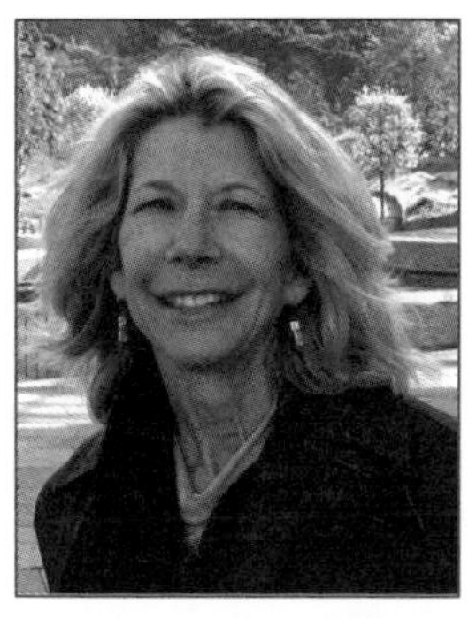

About

Celia Straus

Celia Straus is a writer and nationally known speaker on spiritual parenting and adolescent self-esteem and spirituality. She is the author of two books of spiritual poetry for adolescent girls, *Prayers on My Pillow* and *More Prayers on My Pillow,* as well as *The Mother-Daughter Circle: Making Lifelong Connections with Your Teenager.* Celia holds an MA in English from Georgetown University and is a screenwriter with over 150 top professional awards. She lives in Washington, D.C., with her husband and two daughters. For more information, visit http://exploringwomanhood.com/mindbodysoul/straus/.

In meditation practice, you do not judge what arises in your experience, try to alter it, or engage it in battle. You simply note it without comment in your mind, your emotions, or your body. In that way, you begin to understand that experiences come and go constantly, arising and falling moment by moment, and that even the most solid experiences, such as fear or pain, are fluid in nature.

4

Calming Fear

Judith Lief

The prospect of giving birth and becoming a mother is both exciting and terrifying. From the time we learn we are pregnant until the time we give birth, we experience our lives more intensely than before. So many changes are going on: our body is expanding, our hormone levels are fluctuating, our emotions are heightened, our very definitions of ourselves are changing. At times it can be overwhelming. The phrase "pregnant moment," drawn from the experience of pregnancy, means a time saturated with meaning, overflowing with possibility and with danger.

Every pregnancy is different from every other pregnancy,

so no matter how many stories we have heard from other mothers or how many children we have had, we cannot be sure how a given pregnancy will turn out. We're entering uncertain territory, a place of both hope and fear. In fact, we cycle continuously between hope and fear, doubt and confidence. One moment we imagine we'll be terrible mothers and our children will be deformed; the next moment we think we will be perfect mothers, with perfect, happy children. We live with a mixture of exhilaration and curiosity, not knowing how things will go, how we will do, or who this new being is. Staying with this vulnerability and uncertainty is the best preparation for becoming a mother.

Both hope and fear are based on speculation—what might happen—and on our fixed ideas—what should happen. We want things to go a certain way, we hope all will be well—but we can't be certain. So our hope is paired with fear. Our fear takes the form of what-if thinking. What if something goes wrong? What if I turn out to be a bad mother? What if I don't bond with my child? Though we flip back and forth between hope and fear, by seeing how both arise naturally from our own uncertainty, we can reduce their hold on us. Instead of pretending that everything will be okay or obsessing about what might go wrong, we can learn to ride the waves of hope and fear as they arise—we can note them and let them go. As we do so, we learn to connect with our experience, whatever it may be, with an open heart.

At age thirty I gave birth to my first daughter, Jessica. She arrived five weeks early, and after a long and difficult labor, introduced herself quite straightforwardly. With a penetrating gaze she offered me a glimpse into the powerful yet ungraspable reality from which we spring and to which we return, the realm of boundaries and transitions. At the moment of Jessica's birth, I entered the vast lineage of mothers, those who have held us all in their bodies and brought us into the world. In the same moment that I gave birth to a new child, I gave birth to a new mother. Two years later I gave birth to a second daughter, Deborah, who introduced herself with a friendly glance. Simply and spontaneously, she recognized me and smiled.

As humans we're connected to one another; without such connection we couldn't survive. In particular, we're connected to our mothers. We begin our lives held within our mother, and we must remain there for a while—sheltered within the warmth, protection, and nourishment of her body—if we are to live and grow. But we cannot stay inside forever. To continue to grow, we need to struggle out of our mother and enter the world, alone and vulnerable. Likewise, for a mother to have a child, she must not hold that child within but push it out.

A mother cannot possess her child—if she is to give birth, she must let the child go. And once she does, she cannot control what the child will encounter in his life. She has no choice but to allow the child to enter a world beyond her control, a world that can be unpredictable and dangerous as well as challenging and joyous. On a mother's path, the rhythm of holding and letting go, nurturing and pushing along, is fundamental.

Letting go of expectations is essential, beginning with our expectations about childbirth. A good birth does not always mean a smooth and easy one. Although we may harbor romantic notions of how loving and peaceful we should feel, or how beautiful our birthing experience should be, such romantic scenarios often fall short of the reality of giving birth. For my first child, I had planned a natural childbirth. But five weeks early my water broke, and since labor did not begin on its own, it had to be induced. Since it was a premature labor, it was long and difficult—a scenario that had not been in my plans. I narrowly avoided a Cesarean. For me, giving birth was more gritty than romantic—and much more potent. Like a lotus that rises up from the mud, joy at seeing my daughter blossomed from the experience of reaching my physical and emotional limits.

Giving birth, in fact, is a messy business for any mother. Whether you have a midwife or a doctor, a home birth or a hospital birth, a natural birth or an assisted birth, birth has a physical intensity, involving blood, pain, uncertainty, and risk. It is a physical, mammalian experience, organic, animal, earthy, direct. Yet in that very earthy messiness, as we are pushed to our limits, there's the potential for joy. By joy I don't mean a superficial pleasure that comes and goes and depends on conditions being to our liking. I'm talking about a deeper joy, tinged with sorrow. It is the tender heart of love.

At the moment of birth, the preciousness and immediacy of new life emerging combine with the poignancy and immediacy of our own mortality and that of our child. On the cusps of life, as we enter or leave, we encounter a rawness around the edges. That rawness is nonnegotiable; it has no name; it is bigger than we are—and it inspires awe. All we need to do is surrender to the birthing process, stay with that rawness as we are experiencing it.

How do we prepare ourselves to meet the challenges of birth and motherhood? Like many first-time mothers, before I had my first child, I went to prenatal classes with my husband.

In my class we were taught how to distract ourselves from pain by breathing and by focusing on a point on the wall. But the most useful thing I learned from that class was that pain in one part of the body can cause a cascading of tension in other parts of the body, leading to unnecessary additional pain. I learned to recognize that pattern and to overcome it by relaxing, not by battling the pain or distracting myself from it through various techniques. At the time I took the class, I had already begun to study Buddhism and to practice meditation, or mindfulness-awareness practice, and I found that my experience with simply sitting mindfully and letting experiences arise and fall, moment to moment, was what helped me most.

In meditation practice, you do not judge what arises in your experience, try to alter it, or engage it in battle. You simply note it without comment in your mind, your emotions, or your body. In that way, you begin to understand that experiences come and go constantly, arising and falling moment by moment, and that even the most solid experiences, such as fear or pain, are fluid in nature. The anchor of mindfulness practice is the breath. By placing your attention lightly on the breathing process, you create a kind of space, or room, for whatever your experience is. In that way, instead of being overwhelmed by the intensity of your experience, you learn to accommodate it. When I gave birth to Jessica, I found that changing my perspective from one of avoiding pain to one of allowing room for pain made me better able to handle a long and difficult labor.

Like childbirth, motherhood itself doesn't require us to be perfect, strong, and in control. In fact, trying to be the perfect mom is a trap for both mother and child. Our fixed ideas about how to be mothers put us under enormous pressure. Whatever does not match our expectations is likely to throw us off. And as every mother knows, much of what takes place on the path of motherhood does not match any expectations we might have cooked up. It's like the Hindu story of the great tree and the river grasses. A haughty tree next to a river used to brag to the nearby river grasses about its size and strength. However, when the river flooded, only the big trees were seen tossed out to sea, not the grasses. The river grasses were flexible, so when the floods came, they simply bent and let the water rush by. It's through flexibility, not rigidity, that we thrive.

In the Buddhist tradition, we aspire to treat all sentient beings as our mother, meaning that we show all beings the same love and gratitude we feel toward the person who gave us life and cared for us in childhood. The Buddhist teachings also urge us to love others as a mother loves her only child. A mother puts her child's needs above her own; thus a mother's love represents the highest possibility of love—putting others before self.

It's tempting to view our children as extensions of ourselves, as possessions, or as projects. But if we take this view, we can easily lose our understanding and appreciation for them as they are and instead get caught up in what we want them to become. Thus from the very start, we must let go of our possessiveness and acknowledge our children's separateness from ourselves. If we don't, we either tend to try to smother and control our children or we develop resentment and alienation. Acknowledging our separateness from our children and at the same time appreciating our connection with them form the true underpinnings of parental love.

My children are now grown. Parents and children have only a brief time to spend together. In the end, loving our children means helping them leave and strike out on their own. In the journey from birth to adulthood, I have reflected often on something my teacher, the Tibetan meditation master Chögyam Trungpa Rinpoche, once said—that we should regard our children as honored houseguests. When we invite guests over, we want to share with them the best we have to offer. We clean the house, arrange flowers, set the table, prepare a meal. We anticipate their arrival with pleasure, and when they arrive, we try to make them feel at home by offering them companionship, friendship, and conversation, even though we may have to spend time working behind the scenes while our guests are enjoying themselves. As our guests leave, we thank them for coming and promise to keep in touch. We wave good-bye, close the door, and clean up. We don't consider our guests our possessions. We don't base our identity on them. We don't try to keep them with us forever or mold them in our image. Instead, we value them for their diversity and charm. We invite them in, appreciate them while they're here, share with them the best we have to offer, and send them on their way, well fed and taken care of.

The path of motherhood has a beginning but no end. It's constantly changing and constantly challenging. Along the way, we encounter our personal limits over and over. We fall in love over and over. We ride the sharp edge of hope and fear. On this path of discovery, as on any spiritual path, our pretensions are shattered, our minds are blown, and our hearts are opened. We cry, we laugh, we bumble around and make countless mistakes. Through it all, we are gently—or abruptly—poked into greater honesty, loving-kindness, and understanding. It is a truly joyful path.

PRACTICE

Metta (Loving-kindness) Meditation

CD TRACK 6

Metta is often translated as "loving-kindness." In this practice, we learn to make friends with everyone and everything around us. We begin by extending loving-kindness toward ourselves and our loved ones, and gradually expand the field of metta to include people and things we fear or dislike, and eventually, all beings. One magical aspect of this practice is that as we open our hearts to include things we're afraid of, fear decreases or disappears. Experiment with metta and see if it works this way for you.

There are many ways to practice metta. One way involves saying a series of phrases to ourselves. Traditionally, they are:

May I be free from danger.
May I be happy.
May I be healthy.
May I live with ease.

You can use these if they resonate with you, or you can create new phrases.

We begin metta practice by sitting quietly and directing these phrases to ourselves, silently, for at least a few moments. Then we move on to direct them to someone we love, perhaps our baby.

May you be free from danger.
May you be happy.
May you be healthy.
May you live with ease.

The traditional practice is to then move from someone you love to a "neutral" person, someone whose face or presence you can conjure but who has no personal connection to you. Then we move on to a difficult person and direct the phrases to him or her. You can try it anytime, but it's especially useful when fear and doubt arise.

> *I have a very strong feeling of wanting to really get to know my daughter for who she is. When I was growing up, my mother didn't really seem to know who I was or what I was doing. My intention is to offer my daughter a true companion in addition to a loving mother.*
>
> —Cheryl

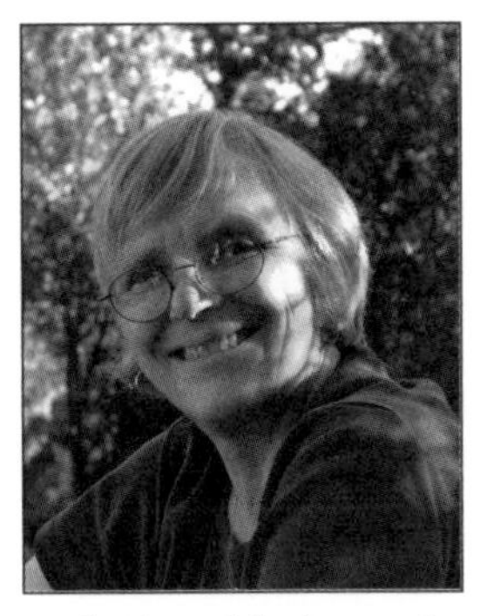

About

Judith Lief

Judith L. Lief has been a Buddhist teacher for over thirty years. She was a close student of Chögyam Trungpa Rinpoche, who trained and empowered her as a teacher in the Buddhist and Shambhala traditions. Sakyong Mipham Rinpoche, his son and successor, recognized Ms. Lief as a senior teacher, or *acharya*. Ms. Lief worked with Trungpa Rinpoche as executive editor of Vajradhatu Publications and from 1980 to 1985 as the dean of Naropa University, in Boulder, Colorado. Currently she is the executive editor of Vajradhatu Publications and the series editor for the Dharma Ocean series, a collection of Trungpa Rinpoche's work published by Shambhala Publications. To learn more about her work, please visit www.judylief.com.

Rituals, traditions, imagination, wonder, and authentic listening can help your child feel a sense of belonging to something grand and good and always available.

We often search for experts to tell us how to be perfect parents, when in fact the answers lie within. Practice following your intuition during pregnancy: "What would taste good to me?" "Should I rest now?" "How does my body want to stretch?" If you heed your inner cues now, intuitive parenting will feel more natural after your baby is born.

5

Setting Intentions

Mimi Doe

I will always recall the day, eleven years ago, when my daughter, Whitney, then a blond-haired sprite of four, and I were sipping lukewarm chamomile tea out of chipped pink plastic teacups on our sunny deck. "I picked you to be my mom," Whitney said out of the blue. "Yup, I was an angel in heaven checking out all the moms, and I said, 'She's the one for me.'"

I was so relieved! If she had picked me to be her mom, then I didn't have to be the all-knowing perfect parent. We were in this dance together, each with her own distinctive identity but joined now as mother and daughter. After hearing Whitney's words, I dropped a big load of control, laughed at my humanness, and began again, knowing that Whitney, the Spirit, and I were on the same page.

Mothering is the ultimate journey of transformation and discovery. During these next months, you have the opportunity to prepare your mind, body, and spirit for this journey.

Once the rhythm of caring for a child begins, you must let go of things like your presumed role, old programming about parenting, fears about being inadequate. You are forced to dissolve into what is—the moment. In the midst of fear and self-doubt, you are sustained simply by drawing on a well of true love. Love keeps you going as it guides and ultimately releases you, whole, to this glorious new relationship with your child.

It's exhilarating to realize that defining the mother role is up to you. You're the grown-up, the mommy, and you may now create a family based on thoughtful, creative, soul-felt intentions. Pregnancy is a wonderful opportunity to consider how you'll nourish your precious child's soul and design for yourself a life lived on purpose.

As you craft your hopes, dreams, and wishes about your mothering role, start by reflecting on how you were mothered. Explore the limitations and gifts you may have inherited from your parents. Just as surely as you will pass on green eyes or black hair, so, too, can you hand these spiritual and emotional traits on to your child. You might begin by drawing a line down the middle of a sheet of paper. On one side, list five gifts you received from your parents—things like time, attention, opportunity, faith. On the other side, list five things your parents did that presented challenges for you. Ask your partner to make his own list, and then combine the two as a starting point for thoughtful discussion about your intentions as parents. In what ways can you help make your child feel accepted, loved, cherished, free, heard, trusted? Asking for wisdom, use your powers of imagination to draw a clear picture of the parent you would like to become. The ever-ready images and promptings will form when you make space for them. Creative visualization helps dissolve barriers and fears, allowing us more easily to manifest our truest selves.

The next step after drawing a picture of yourself as a mother is to craft a soul relationship with your child. Your child is not separate from you—she is physically connected to you now and will be emotionally and spiritually connected to you for both of your lifetimes. And yet this child has her own path, her own unfolding destiny. Giving birth seems to be about allowing a soulful relationship to grow without grasping the strings of control.

To counter images of yourself as a parent who sacrifices your identity for this baby, reflect on a fulfilling relationship you have experienced. You'll most likely notice that it's what you bring of your authentic self to this relationship that ultimately makes it so satisfying. After all, a real relationship is one in which you are seen, heard, honored, and known as your unique self. Yes, it's important to read mothering self-help books and carefully heed your doctor's instructions for caregiving. But beyond all this lies the truth of two people in a relationship, two people who need to find their way to each other with grace, truth, and love. You will be so much more than simply a caregiver—your presence and spirit matter more than your tasks and obligations. Thus, you will want to explore deeply and learn to fill your own well so that you can bring more of yourself, edges more clearly defined, to this relationship with your son or daughter.

Finally, along with taking prenatal vitamins, preparing the nursery, and reading up on child development, try some of the following mindful mothering exercises to prepare for the arrival of your baby:

- Cultivate time alone to dream, plan, and tune in to the rhythm of the new life within you. The changes in your body urge you to take a break from your normal routine and offer a powerful opportunity to align yourself with your inner world. Try the meditations included on this book's CD and the journaling exercises at the end of this chapter.

- One of the joys of pregnancy is all the positive remarks both friends and strangers share with you. It's as if the world is conspiring to bolster you with love. As you prepare to mother, open your heart to receive more love from your partner, parents, friends, pets, and coworkers. Imagine yourself taking all this nourishing energy and wrapping it around you and your baby as a cocoon of warm, gentle light.

- None of us is perfect, and this is especially true for parents. Thus, letting go takes on a whole new meaning from here on. Begin to practice releasing unrealistic expectations of yourself. You are growing a new life—a monumental job—so go easy on yourself. There will be no grade at the end of these nine months, no promotion, no gold star. Instead there will be a new life that you've cocreated, a miracle you've been privileged to harbor.

- Become aware of your inner treasures and how you might express them through family life, moment by moment. Practice bringing yourself fully to ordinary activities: lathering your growing tummy with lotion, setting the table for dinner, selecting nourishing music for the drive to work, and so on. The creative spiritual call of mother is "Be here, be here now"—and eventually "Be here, see me, honor me, join me in this moment, Mom!"

- Mothering is a rich and creative activity. Fostering and nourishing your child's spirit is as creative an endeavor as writing a novel or painting a masterpiece. Opportunities to explore this kind of creativity will present themselves each day. You can put your toddler in front of a television—or an easel. You can give your baby a bath with your hands while your mind sorts through the data needed for an upcoming talk, or you can listen fully to the squeals of delight or cries of discomfort and take in the smell of sweet baby skin.

- We often search for experts to tell us how to be perfect parents, when in fact the answers lie within. Practice following your intuition during pregnancy: "What would taste good to me?" "Should I rest now?" "How does my body want to stretch?" If you heed your inner cues now, intuitive parenting will feel more natural after your baby is born.

- Begin to create spiritual meaning for yourself. Don't wait to find just the right church, temple, or spiritual practice. Many parents ask questions like "Should we baptize? Should we circumcise? Should we go to services each week? How can we choose between our two religions?" I can't answer these questions for you, but I can tell you that courageously taking action to articulate and claim your family's unique set of spiritual beliefs paves the way for the unfolding of a shared sacred identity. Every family needs spiritual grounding, every day of the week. Rituals, traditions, imagination, wonder, and authentic listening can help your child feel a sense of belonging to something grand and good and always available.

- Release the notion that your child will fulfill your every expectation: think instead of how you might fulfill your own expectations of yourself as a mother.

Becoming a parent is filled with possibilities. Your quest is to remain open to the miraculous discoveries both you and your child can make every day.

Blessings and light from my heart to yours on this mystical, marvelous mothering journey.

PRACTICE

Journaling

Reflecting in writing on your values as a parent can lend enormous help and clarity to your parenting. Try writing in your journal on some of the following topics, either on your own or with your partner.

The five most valuable things I received from my parents were . . .

The five things I learned from my parents that I still find myself trying to undo are . . .

If I could magically impart three core values to my child, they would be . . . . Why those three?

The three things I'm most afraid my child will learn from me are . . .

The three things I most hope my child will learn from me are . . .

To parent well, you have to have the gentleness and courage of a warrior.

—Carol

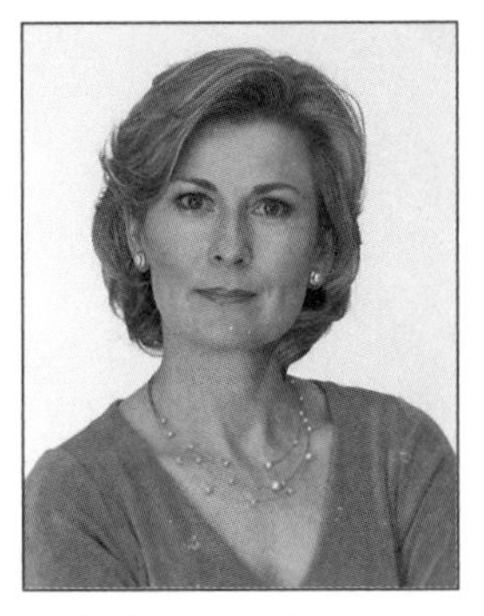

About

Mimi Doe

Mimi Doe has authored five books on parenting and families and has won the Parents' Choice Seal of Approval for *10 Principles for Spiritual Parenting. Ladies' Home Journal* has called Mimi "a parenting guru," and her work has been covered in publications such as *Child, Parenting, McCall's, Family Circle, Publishers Weekly,* and *USA Today.* She has appeared on *The Oprah Winfrey Show.* She holds a master's degree in education from Harvard and has presented life-changing workshops to parenting groups, churches, educational conferences, and professional associations. Her popular online newsletter, "Spiritual Parenting Thought for the Week," has over fifty thousand subscribers from around the world, and parents have begun Spiritual Parenting groups to focus on Doe's clear principles.

For more tips and ideas from Mimi, visit www.spiritualparenting.com.

When all other schemes and devices fall away, the breath is all we have to use. It never fails us. Pregnancy is a good time to get to know your breath, through simple awareness practices such as meditation and yoga. While sitting, lying down, walking, or moving, bringing your attention to your belly and the natural movement of the breath will strengthen your connection to your own life force, the awareness that is ever-present and unafraid.

6

Preparing for Childbirth

Karen Maezen Miller

Of course you want to be prepared.

You want to know what is best for your child—during pregnancy and ever after—the studies, the findings, and the expert recommendations. On issues this large and lasting, you want to know where to stand, and so you prepare. Anyone would.

You want to do what is right, driven by a current of incomparable love and overwhelming uncertainty. You want to have no regrets, and so you prepare.

You want to graciously receive the wisdom of those who have gone before, and honor the impulse of your own maternal choices. You want to do it your way, and so you prepare.

But by the anxious later stages of pregnancy, and in the dazed early weeks of new motherhood, you may begin to doubt that any of that was ever possible. You may no longer believe that you have learned enough, done enough, or prepared enough. Who could?

You. You can believe that you are prepared.

No matter what you have or haven't done, you have prepared. Visibly and invisibly, life always prepares itself, and in this way, you are prepared for the very things you might never have expected. I learned this myself, and you will learn it too. All mothers learn it, through the inconceivable experience of pregnancy and childbirth, experiences that propel us beyond fearful delusions and into our own abiding source of wisdom.

I was seven months pregnant when I walked into my doctor's office for my scheduled checkup and said what I had been afraid to admit for weeks. "I don't feel well."

"You have preeclampsia," the doctor said, after a urine test and blood pressure check confirmed my worst fears. "Go to the hospital right now."

Around five percent of expectant mothers develop what I had: hypertension, swelling, and protein in the urine, symptoms that the body is rejecting the placenta. There are grave and even fatal consequences to the untreated sufferer. Deliver the child and preeclampsia goes away.

My picture-perfect pregnancy was over. All my plans were obsolete. My good intentions were for naught; my high standards, shot. I was lucky for the late onset of the disease: odds favored my baby's health. Even so, it was hard to judge the outcome as anything but total failure. I must have done something terribly wrong! Where was the misstep, the error, or the omission? Like most of the fears I harbored about my body, my mind, my baby, and myself, these were misplaced. Fear is always the result of misplaced focus.

There is an unexpected end to every pregnancy. The end is the birth itself, and whether early or late, easy or difficult, every birth is unpredictable and astonishing. Pregnancy prepares us as all of life prepares us. It prepares us to let go of how we thought it would be, and to focus on how it is. It prepares us to dwell solely on what appears in front of us, instead of on the anxious, fearful ruminations in our head. No matter how you think or feel, you can literally *see* how prepared you are already, and you can trust it.

You are prepared by your body. I can faintly remember the terror and awe I felt as my body ballooned to bursting over the course of my pregnancy. Awe, because I did nothing. Terror, because *I did nothing*, at least not in the way I had usually done things, with the force of an iron will and a zest for managing details. Suffice it to say, I was accustomed to being in charge. In no area of my life was I afraid of doing what needed to be done—taking the lead, calling the shots—and here was the most ambitious project, the veritable mother of all makeovers, and I was, for all practical purposes, sidelined by sleepiness, hunger, discomfort, distraction, and immobility, even before I was kicked out of the cockpit by a medical emergency.

So it is. Pregnancy has a life of its own. Even in normal circumstances it proceeds without our input as we widen, thicken, fill, bulge, stretch, spread, and then literally split from one whole body and heart into two. To be sure, we take our vitamins, try to eat well, and exercise, but who can even imagine the undertaking? Who can plan, diagram, analyze, and control it? No one, and no one needs to, since the mystery of life is self-revealed. With or without complications, pregnancy is preparation for the miraculous breakthrough of birth and the immeasurable expansion of life and love that comes after. It prepares us for all that by taking it out of our hands.

In all honesty, I can recall pregnancy and birth only faintly because of one other marvel for which we are ingeniously prepared: to forget every bit of it. A mother's mind is reengineered to forget what is best forgotten, and to remember everything else.

You are prepared by your mind. It's not just in your head. You're different. Hormones change the brain during pregnancy to prepare you for the most important relationship of your life—and to help you adapt to new levels of learning, mental stress, physical exertion, and emotional intimacy. You become more resilient, attentive, and intuitive. You have entered an experience beyond the reach of logic and reason, farther than the limits of anything you can comprehend. At times, you may think you've lost your mind, and that may be part of it. Still, without knowing how, you will most certainly know best. How do I know? Mothers always know best. Now you can breathe easier.

You are prepared by your breath. Just this one little thing, the breath, delivers all the wisdom in the world. Each inhalation powers your strength, endurance, and concentration; each exhalation releases your resistance and fears. Birth gives testament to the miracle of the breath, and yet, do we really know what the breath is?

I had practiced meditation for years before my pregnancy, realizing the benefits of mental clarity and quietude by simply bringing my attention to the natural flow of the breath. When we bring our agitated minds into focus by following the movement of the breath in and out of the body, we experience the reality of the present moment, free from confusion and anxiety. The breath is fearlessness personified. That can matter a great deal to you in the pain and panic of childbirth, as well as in the anxiety that precedes it. How wonderful that all the sages and wise women, the birth educators and coaches, the doulas and midwives, tell you to breathe! Focusing on the breath is the safest, surest way to overcome fear and let the immediacy of any experience move forward.

"Use your practice," my Zen teacher reminded me on the eve of my labor induction. When all other schemes and devices fall away, the breath is all we have to use. It never fails us. Pregnancy is a good time to get to know your breath, through simple awareness practices such as meditation and yoga. While sitting, lying down, walking, or moving, bringing your attention to your belly and the natural movement of the breath will strengthen your connection to your own life force, the awareness that is ever-present and unafraid. The breath will not only transport you beyond fear, it will deliver you to joy. In the flow of the breath, the mother and child come into being, and joy springs to life.

You are prepared by your joy. From the first moment you knew you were expecting, and in the smile, the glow, the giddy laughter, and the inexplicable tears—you have been prepared by joy. What is joy? It is not one certain thing or feeling, not even one sensation or experience. Joy is the radiating fullness of life itself: surprising, delightful, natural, and, beneath all the words that fail to name it, simply good. Life is good, and joy is the gift born to those who know life's goodness.

I can't tell you where joy comes from, but I can tell you when. Joy comes the moment you open your disbelieving eyes and weary arms to receive it. You will know joy a half second after giving birth, when you hold your newborn to your bosom and you and the baby both sob in bleary recognition. You will find joy in the exquisitely perfect face; silky touch; soothing warmth, sound, and smell of your baby—yes, every one of those sounds and smells, every time. You will take joy in the deep dark of a long night when an inconsolable cry finally quiets and vanishes into the mists of instant slumber, and you watch, grateful and silent, as peace descends like a blanket into the soft shadows around you. You will greet joy in the morning, at the first crack of your child's beaming smile, a coo, and a giggle.

Life will suddenly be so funny, so sweet, so precious, so

very much of everything! Joy is life, uncontained and effervescent. You will be endlessly filled by joy, but you cannot keep it. What you can hold on to is not joy but fear, and fear is preparing you too.

You are prepared by your fear. But wait, you say, I am still so afraid! Yes, you most certainly are afraid and it's okay to be afraid, because your fear is preparing you to be unafraid. You are being schooled in the rarefied and often irrational powers of discernment: to detect and deflect unseen risks, to read signs and labels, to guess and then second-guess, to wait, to hear and heed warnings, and to courageously move forward. Fear need never be hidden or denied, but faced bare in the bright openness of tender respect and patience. Given its voice, fear asks for help, and then takes the help that comes, because fear prepares you to trust what you do not yet know and cannot see: what will happen next.

You are prepared by your trust. What is the outcome of this extraordinary experience called "expecting," an outcome that may not have occurred when you'd planned, proceeded as you'd hoped, or culminated in the slightest sense of self-certainty? The outcome is trust, the same trust that will carry you along in all the days and nights ahead. Trust is a mother's companion—her most faithful and trustworthy one.

With the trust you already have in your bones, your blood, and your breath, you can trust your own confusion as the parent of clarity, your own doubt as the mother of confidence.

You can trust that even if the path veers off the map, the way will always be clear.

You can trust family and friends, and trust strangers to become friends.

You can trust time and the inevitability of change. You can trust that when you think you can't handle it for one more minute, you can handle it for one more minute.

You can trust your strength, courage, and flexibility; you can trust your body in ways you never dreamed of.

You can trust your child. You can trust yourself.

You will lose trust, and then find trust again. Many, many times.

You can trust in every outcome. You can trust in your life as it unfolds. Prepared or not, you can trust, because your life has prepared you to be awake, attentive, receptive, attuned, and responsive to whatever occurs. You have been prepared to be unprepared. This is the paradox of pregnancy and the magnificence of which you are now the heir and incarnation. This is what makes you a mother.

You are prepared to be unprepared. When my tiny daughter

came home from the hospital nearly two weeks after her premature birth, there was not one thing lacking in our preparation, and yet nothing had gone according to plan.

I can promise the same is true for you. You have everything you need, and what you don't yet have will arrive as surely as your next breath. You have been chosen. You have been groomed. You have been readied by your waiting, and taught by the quickening pulse of your brimming heart. Any day now, you can stop expecting, focus your body, mind, and breath on the moment at hand, and leap into the fearless wonder of the unplanned life.

You can believe it, because you can believe in yourself.

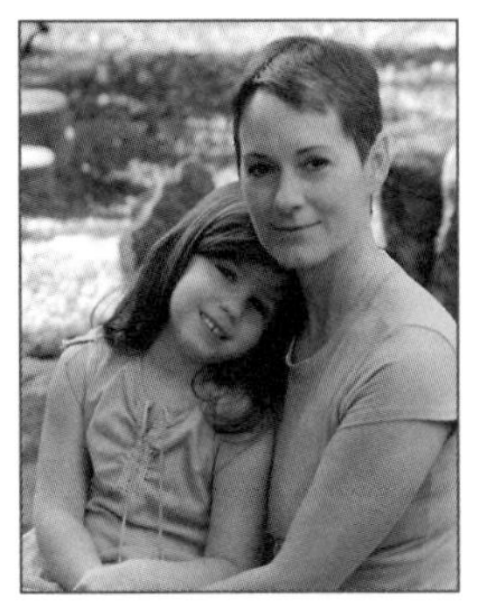

About

Karen Maezen Miller

Karen Maezen Miller is a wife and mother as well as a Zen Buddhist priest and teacher, or *sensei,* at the Hazy Moon Zen Center in Los Angeles. She and her family live in Sierra Madre, California, with a century-old Japanese garden in their backyard. She is the author of *Momma Zen: Walking the Crooked Path of Motherhood* and *Hand Wash Cold: Care Instructions for an Ordinary Life.* For more information on her work, retreats, and other events, please visit www.karenmaezenmiller.com.

Dedication of Merit

It is traditional to dedicate any good that may have arisen from our spiritual practice to the benefit of all beings. This way, we are practicing for the whole world, not just ourselves. You may use your own words to indicate your intention to practice for the benefit of all beings, or you may recite this Jewel Heart sangha translation of the Four Immeasurables:

> May all beings have happiness and the causes of happiness.
> May all beings be free from suffering and the causes of suffering.
> May all beings never be parted from freedom's true joy.
> May all beings dwell in equanimity, free from attachment and aversion.

Resources

Books and CDs by Contributors to *The Mindful Way through Pregnancy*

Anne Cushman

From Here to Nirvana (Riverhead Books)

Mimi Doe

Busy but Balanced: Practical and Inspirational Ways to Create a Calmer, Closer Family (St. Martin's Griffin)

Drawing Angels Near: Children Tell of Angels in Words and Pictures (Atria Books)

10 Principles for Spiritual Parenting: Nurturing Your Child's Soul (with Marsha Walch, PhD) (HarperCollins)

Judith Lief

Making Friends with Death: A Buddhist Guide to Encountering Mortality (Shambhala Publications)

The Heart of the Buddha by Chögyam Trungpa (Judith Lief, editor) (Shambhala Publications)
Training the Mind by Chögyam Trungpa (Judith Lief, editor) (Shambhala Publications)

Celia Straus

I'm More Than What I Seem (audio CD) (Padma Projects)
Prayers on My Pillow: Inspiration for Girls on the Threshold of Change (Ballantine)
More Prayers on My Pillow: Words of Comfort and Hope for Girls on the Journey to Self (Ballantine)
The Mother-Daughter Circle: Making Lifelong Connections with Your Teenager (Ballantine)

Karen Maezen Miller

Momma Zen: Walking the Crooked Path of Motherhood (Shambhala Publications)
Hand Wash Cold: Care Instructions for an Ordinary Life (New World Library)

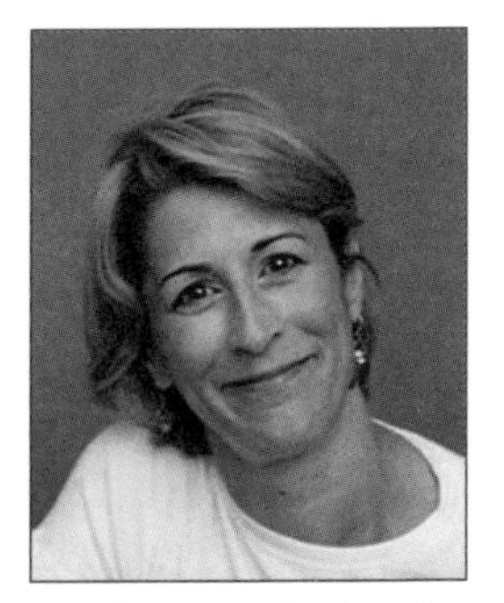

About Susan Piver

Susan Piver is an author, meditation teacher, and the founder and creative director of Padma Media, which creates projects that support an awakened life. Her latest effort is the Open Heart Project, which delivers guided meditation instruction and insights to your inbox.

You can read more about Susan Piver at http://susanpiver.com.

CD Track List

The Mindful Way through Pregnancy,
Meditation Instructions

Led by Susan Piver

1. Introduction	0:31
2. Introduction to the Practices	1:26
3. Basic Breath Awareness	9:56
4. Body Awareness Meditation	8:54
5. Sending and Taking Meditation	7:32
6. Metta (Loving-kindness) Meditation	9:28